HEART
LIFESTYLE &

Cardiac problems and those ailments owing to high blood pressure occupy the top of the list among the major causes of death and disability in adults. Many people, mostly men, succumb to the fatal stroke of a heart attack at the prime of their life when they are most creative and productive in their career. Though rapid, scientific developments in the last fifty years in some advanced countries have helped in bringing down the death rates occurring from heart attacks, in most of the developing world, cardiac diseases still pose a major challenge to life and longevity. A curative approach to heart diseases is turning out to be very expensive both for the family as well as for the state. The riddle of the cause of heart attacks yet remains unsolved. Since this disease is multifactorial in nature, hence its control, prevention and management have to be multipronged. Lifestyle has a major role in the cause and cure of many modern diseases including heart attacks. This book focuses on the interrelationship of lifestyle, prevention of heart disease and the role of modern drugs and devices in attaining longevity through optimum heart care.

Padmashri Dr Harbans Singh Wasir (MD, DM, FAMS, FNASc) is Professor and Head of the Department of Cardiology at the All India Institute of Medical Sciences, New Delhi. Having joined the AIIMS in 1957 as an undergraduate, Prof. Wasir has had a brilliant academic career spanning through his first position in Medicine, and over 350 scientific publications in international and national medical journals and six books related to heart care to his credit. He has travelled widely to participate in scientific medical conferences, besides being a visiting professor to the Universities of Leuven, Belgium and Gothenburg, Sweden. Recipient of several national awards including the Dr. B.C. Roy Award for research in medicine, the Indian Council of Medical Research Award in Cardiology, and several citations for his notable contribution in Cardiology, Prof. Wasir is also a consultant to the Indian Armed Forces and World Health Organisation. He's an honorary physician to the President of India.

By the same author

1. Heart to Heart — A Holistic Approach to Heart Care
2. Aging and Heart Care
3. Heart Management — A Manual for Promotive and Preventive Heart Care
4. Haardik Samvad (Hindi)
5. Traditional Wisdom for Heart Care
6. Preventive Cardiology — An Introduction
7. *Dil Tn'o Dilan´ Lei* (Punjabi)

Published by
Sterling Publishers Private Limited

HEART CARE
LIFESTYLE & LONGEVITY

DR. H. S. WASIR
MD, DM, FAMS, FNASc

Professor & Head, Dept. of Cardiology
All India Institute of Medical Sciences

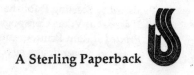

A Sterling Paperback

STERLING PAPERBACKS
An imprint of
Sterling Publishers (P) Ltd.
L-10, Green Park Extension, New Delhi-110016
Ph.: 6511784, 6511785 Fax: 91-11-6851028

HEART CARE: Lifestyle & Longevity
©1997, Dr. H.S. Wasir
ISBN 81 207 1946 8
Reprint 1997

All rights are reserved. No part of this publication may be reproduced, stored in a retrieval system or transmitted, in any form or by any means, mechanical, photocopying, recording or otherwise, without prior written permission of the publisher.

Published by Sterling Publishers Pvt. Ltd., New Delhi-110016.
Laserset at Vikas Compographics, New Delhi-110029.
Printed at Ram Printograph (India), New Delhi-110020.
Cover design by Narendra Vashishta

Dedicated
to
all those who give love and warmth
to others, making life meaningful
and worth living.

CONTENTS

	Foreword	ix
	Preface	xi
	Prologue	xv
1.	Common Heart Problems and Their Management	1
2.	Mind and Heart	10
3.	Lifestyle and Longevity	20
4.	Diet, Alcohol, Smoking and Exercise	30
5.	Blood Pressure—High and Low	51
6.	Environmental Pollution, Heart Diseases and Longevity	57
7.	Role of the Spouse in Heart Care	68
8.	Drugs, Devices and Devotion in Heart Care	76
9.	Ayurveda and Heart Care	84
10.	Yoga and the Heart	90
11.	Old Age, Modern Medicine and Longevity	98
	Epilogue	110
	Glossary of Medical Terms	111
	Index	115

FOREWORD

I welcome the publication of Professor Wasir's book: *Heart Care - Lifestyle and Longevity*. It shows the overriding importance of health promotion, not only based on the findings of newer research studies, but also based on the traditional wisdom as reflected in the ancient scripts of India. This wide-ranging view from ancient scripts to the most modern and sophisticated diagnostic and therapeutic interventions lends a truly holistic purview of cardiovascular diseases and their prevention and control, which should make a fascinating reading. The publication comes at a time when South-East Asia is witnessing a slow but steady increase in cardiovascular diseases.

The book's strength arises from its down-to-earth approach to one of the major concerns of modern health professions and health planners alike, viz., the merging issue of healthy and happy aging.

Dr. Uton Muchtar Rafei
Regional Director
World Health Organisation
South East Asia Region, New Delhi

PREFACE

My first book, *Heart to Heart — A Holistic Approach to Heart Care* published in 1990, was dedicated to "Physicians, Poets and Physiologists; Singers, Scholars and Spiritualists — who are involved with the well-being of human heart". This dedication was based on my observations over the years that the human heart is much more than merely a muscular pump pushing blood for the body needs. Even when other organs may be having a little siesta, the heart goes on working nonstop, like a sentinel on perennial duty, guarding the awake and the asleep alike. The internal environment of our body called the "milieu interior" is no doubt important for the physiological normal functioning of the heart, but equally important for the well-being of the human heart is the external environment including the diet we eat, the air we breathe, the provocative people we meet and the stressful situations we face in our day to day living. It is because of this multifaceted situation that the human heart is associated with and the fact that we, as yet, do not know the exact cause of heart attacks, that the last book I wrote was entitled, *Traditional Wisdom for Heart Care*, in which I further extended the concept of holistic heart care.

Human longevity is being affected adversely by a change in people's lifestyles through their faulty eating habits (heart diseases, hypertension, diabetes, obesity and cancer), permissiveness in sexual habits (AIDS), tobacco consumption (lung cancer, other lung diseases and heart attacks) and addiction to alcohol and life-threatening drugs (mental aberration, cognitive disorders, homicidal and suicidal tendencies and accidental deaths). These diseases altogether are responsible for the major mortality and morbidity in the adults in most countries of the world in whatever social or economic category you place them. These so-called lifestyle-related diseases obviously are due to our own making and not the will of God. Hence, it has to be through our own efforts that we should be able to control, prevent and possibly eradicate most of these diseases, thereby ensuring a productive long life to the members of this global family of human race.

In the present book, I have focused on the subject of longevity through proper heart care, as it is through heart attacks, high blood pressure and brain attacks (stroke) that life is being cut short in millions of adults, and in many of those who survive these attacks, they lead only a sub-optimal life instead of being "full of life". Although modern drugs, intervention devices and surgical wonders have given a new lease of life to many, yet the curative treatment for cardiovascular diseases by ballooning, laser, stents and bypass surgery is prohibitively expensive and beyond the reach of many families. The state budget also does not provide for such costly treatment and the medical insurance for majority of population in India and many other countries is non-existent. Prevention of heart diseases and hypertension should be through hygienic measures, lifestyle modifications, and non-drug means, such as: (1) Balanced diet comprising more vegetables and fruits menu than dairy products and meats. Total diet intake should be restricted so as not to become fat. (2) Avoiding excess salt and alcohol consumption. (3) Prohibiting the use of tobacco in any form. (4) Avoiding sedentary lifestyle and doing physical exercises regularly. (5) Facing stressful situations with a positive attitude and adopting ways and means to get mental relaxation through study of religious texts, music, meditation and yoga.

If a periodic check-up reveals a person having high blood pressure, diabetes or high blood lipids like cholesterol, triglycerides, etc., one should not hesitate to start appropriate drug therapy to keep the blood pressure, blood sugar and blood lipids in normal range. Normalising blood lipids and blood pressure result in lowering the occurrence of heart attacks. There are potent drugs available for all these disorders and one must make use of these when required, but under periodic monitoring for their side-effects and under close supervision of the physician. Apart from the potent drugs for treatment and prevention of various heart diseases, we have at present most advanced intervention devices such as angioplasty, stents, pacemakers, radio frequency ablations, and automatic cardiac defibrillators, etc., for treatment of most of the heart ailments and for prevention of recurrence of heart attacks and other events related to cardiovascular disorders. All these therapeutic measures have, in fact, not only made the lives of victims of heart disease free from pain and other symptoms, but have certainly saved many from dying prematurely, thereby prolonging their longevity and improving the quality of life. These aspects of heart care through lifestyles, drugs, devices and surgical measures, in the treatment of those with heart disease and preventing its recurrence, and for primary prevention or postponement of heart attacks to the age beyond three scores plus ten, have been highlighted in the present book. Hopefully, the book will help in giving this message of heart care to the masses through the medium of physicians, parents and public interaction. These timely preventive measures and therapeutic interventions with modern drugs, devices and surgical techniques will prevent more and more people from dying prematurely and thus living longer and productive lives.

The price for this crusade of writing books on several facets of heart care and the numerous public lectures and newspaper articles on related topics, has been rather high for me. This has been in the form of being away from the family on most weekends and holidays and even when at home, not being on speaking terms with anyone and staying in my study den under self-imposed quarantine. I hope, Jasjeet, Harpreet, Kamalpreet and Bhupender will forgive me for this lapse, but at the same time, being themselves in the medical profession they will understand and ought to be prepared for such experiences among the fraternity. In medical profession, it is our commitment and devotion, beyond our usual duty for treatment of the sick, to disseminate the message of prevention of disease, preserving and promoting health. The present book is an effort in this direction concerning heart care.

Harbans S. Wasir

PROLOGUE

Dr. H.S. Wasir has been a crusader, a missionary who not only treats the ill, but has made it a mission of his life to educate the common man in preventing heart disease, and guide the ailing how to manage, improve the quality of life and even prolong it. Starting with his first book, *Heart to Heart - A Holistic Approach to Heart Care,* in 1990, he has been producing a book a year on broadly the same subject. This is besides his frequent articles in the daily newspapers and magazines, and of course, scientific contributions in academic journals, which have been recognised by the scientific community, resulting in the conferment of a prestigious Fellowship of the National Academy of Sciences on him. Having spent a lifetime working at the All India Institute of Medical Sciences, I know Cardiology is one of the busiest departments with a very heavy service load. I am amazed at Dr. Wasir's output in spite of devoting long hours to his patients.

Coronary heart disease was generally believed to be much more prevalent in the Western society than in the developing countries like the Indian subcontinent. But it has been proved to be a myth as the current epidemiological studies have shown. Our population is paying the price for its development, the high-voltage living, adoption of Western mores and atmospheric pollution, an avoidable accompaniment of haphazard industrialisation. Heart disease is preventively manageable but not radically curable. This is Dr. Wasir's crusade — to educate the common man, how he can avoid paying the price with his health and heart for development, as our society yearns to evolve from the have-nots to the haves among the people of the world. And if he has the disease, which has a tendency of being often inherited, how he can avoid its complications, manage it within limits and live not only meaningfully, but enjoy his life and even prolong it.

The author has made a deep study of our scriptures and ancient texts on health care. He has pulled out pearls of ancient wisdom from *Charaka Samhita* (600 BC) and *Patanjali* (300 BC) on health care which are as applicable today as they were in the past — as quoted here in the chapters on Yoga and Ayurveda and Heart Care. It is truly amazing how accurate are the descriptions of the malfunctions of the heart, like disorders of rhythm in those ancient texts and how applicable, their prescriptions were to prevent complications, and keep cardiac disorders under control, as judged by our current knowledge. What Dean Ornish is prescribing today was what our ancient texts did centuries ago in the management of heart disease and its complications, like the importance of meditation, relaxation, Yogic exercises and moderation in eating and, in fact, our lifestyle. The control of mind over the health of the heart as described in those texts was as emphasized by William Harvey in the seventeenth century and as we know today.

In this book, Dr. Wasir has again covered the entire gamut of coronary heart disease in a layman's language starting with imparting awareness on common heart problems and their management, the role of lifestyle, diet, alcohol and smoking, the place of drugs and devices. An interesting and useful chapter is on the role of spouse and health care — the part it plays in aggravating or assuaging heart disease. The book ends with a note of cheer and advice for the old and aging with a very appropriate keynote that "Age has more to do with your attitudes and thoughts than the biological aging alone" and a fitting finale in the verse by Longfellow.

On the whole, the book makes an easy reading — a useful health guide and a recipe for a more enjoyable living while tending the most crucial asset of the human body.

Prof. H.D. Tandon
Former Director
All India Institute of Medical Sciences
New Delhi.

1
COMMON HEART PROBLEMS AND THEIR MANAGEMENT

Let us cherish and love old age; for it is full of pleasure, if one knows how to use it.... The best morsel is reserved to the last.
— SENECA, *Epistular ad Lucilium.* Epis. xii, sec. 4.

Whether it is a hospital, hotel, household or any hi-tech industrial establishment, we're living in an era of management. Doing graduation or masters, business management is the most sought after vocation of the day. It is this need of the hour that has seen many institutions of business management, including hotel and hospital management, emerging and flourishing both in the government and private sectors over the last three decades or so. Well-planned management strategies form the keyword for most of the successful organisations, individuals and nations.

Drawing upon the same analogy, heart being the most important organ of our body, it needs the utmost care for its well-being and proper functioning for our health and longevity. It is like the engine of your car. As any loose nut or bolt, clogged fuel pipe, particulate matter in the carburator or short-circuiting of wiring system will put the car out of action, same is the story with heart. Management strategies for car care apply to heart care as well, i.e. (a) *Preventive strategies* and (b) *Curative strategies* to be followed in case of its breakdown. Like a periodic, regular check-up services for the car engine is the preventive approach for heart care involving lifestyle measures, which include nutritional aspects, doing regular physical exercise, avoiding smoking and practice of techniques that bring mental relaxation such as meditation, yoga, music and attending religious congregations. These preventive and promotive measures for heart care have often been talked and written about under the banner of lifestyles and will be dealt with in detail in subsequent chapters. But right now, let's straight away get down to the curative and corrective measures to be taken in case of any breakdown of this toughest organ in our body, the heart, that goes on working nonstop for decades together and at times even crosses a century. A commendable task indeed!

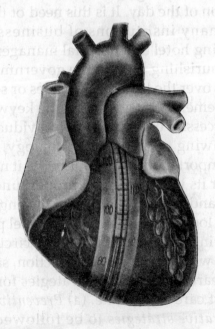

Heart Defects and Their Management

The various defects that take this machine (heart) to the workshop (hospital) comprise the following:

1) Certain holes and blocks present from birth, disturbing and diverting the blood flow in wrong directions.
2) Disorders of the valves due to rheumatic fever and rheumatic heart disease.
3) Clogged coronary arteries that supply fuel (oxygenated blood) for this engine, i.e., the heart, giving rise to anginal pain and heart attacks.
4) Getting fatigued and weak because of having overworked for long hours under undue pressure, i.e., heart disease due to high blood pressure (hypertension).
5) Defective wiring system (conduction system) resulting in disorders of heartbeat and irregular rhythm (arrhythmia).
6) Flabby heart muscles disease (cardiomyopathy) due to excessive alcohol, infections, diabetes and other systemic diseases.

Miscellaneous Defects

Certain disorders of other organs or systems in the body may adversely affect this engine—like thyroid malfunction, both underactivity (hypothyroidism) or overactivity (hyperthyroidism), anemia, malnutrition and systemic infections, specially tuberculosis which affects the outer covering of the heart — pericardium (pericarditis).

Alarm Signals of Heart Trouble

Basically there are four cardinal signals (symptoms) that make us suspect and bring the person with heart disease to see a physician. These are (1) Chest pain (2) Palpitation (3) Breathlessness and (4) Fatigue.

1. Chest Pain

One of the many causes of chest pain is heart trouble. It is the type and description of pain that distinguishes the cardiac pain from other non-cardiac causes of chest pain. Central chest pain, radiating to either or both arms, more often the left arm, lasting from a few minutes to half an hour or so, associated with a feeling of constriction in chest or heaviness, is often the description of pain due to heart disease. Non-cardiac causes of chest pain include cervical spondylosis, peptic ulcer, gall bladder disease, herpes and anemia. The commonest cause of cardiac chest pain (angina and myocardial infarction) is the narrowing of coronary arteries (coronary artery disease) due to the process called atherosclerosis. The aggravating risk factors for this disease are high blood cholesterol, smoking and high blood pressure. Patients having blocked coronary arteries can be successfully treated these days with the help of potent drugs such as nitrates, beta and calcium blocker, ACE (Angiotensin Converting Enzyme) inhibitors and aspirin. Ballooning by angioplasty, atherectomy and using stents (small wire coils) to keep the dilated arteries patent, are some of the non-surgical means to take effective care of pain due to coronary artery disease.

These measures definitely improve the exercise performance and quality of life of such patients with coronary disease. Bypass surgery using veins and artery conduits has revolutionised the management strategies for patients with coronary artery disease, giving them not only an angina-free improved quality of life but also more longevity. Presently, there is an additional help available from TMR (Transmyocardial Laser Revascularisation) in those patients who have very poor left ventricular ejection power and not too good graftable arteries.

Anginal pain can also be due to narrowed or leaky heart valves, specially the aortic valve. Replacement or repair of the diseased valves is the surgical treatment for such maladies.

2. Palpitation

It is the uncomfortable awareness of one's heartbeat. Normally one is not aware of the continuous beating of heart, even during exercise, but in certain diseased states an uncomfortable awareness occurs and that brings the person to a hospital or a physician for heart check-up. Causes of palpitation may be non-cardiac also, like anemia, thyrotoxicosis and rarely during pregnancy. The cardiac causes of palpitation include rheumatic heart disease with obstructive or leaky valves, congenital cardiac defects and disorders of conduction system of heart, called arrhythmias. Both fast heartbeat and very slow heartbeat can give rise to palpitation. Skipped or missing beats or extra but weak heartbeats also manifest as a disagreeable sensation in the chest. Management approach for palpitation is directed towards the cause, like surgical repair or replacement of defective heart valves, ballooning the narrow stenotic valves (valvoplasty), use of various potent antiarrhythmic drugs, radio-frequency energy to ablate abnormal focus of cardiac contraction, implanting of cardiac pacemakers and Intracardiac Cardioverter Defibrillators (ICD). The latter device (ICD), has helped to prevent recurrence of fatal arrhythmias in survivors of sudden cardiac death, who survived after resuscitation measures.

3. Breathlessness

In the event of breathing difficulty, one is likely to think of lung problems, but breathlessness may occur often, not only during work or exertion but at times also at rest due to diseases of heart. The reason for this symptom in heart patients is pooling of blood and raised pressure in the pulmonary circuit (lungs), due to narrowed or leaking valves in the left-sided chambers of the heart that either receive blood from the lungs (mitral valve) or eject out blood to the body (aortic valve). Breathlessness also occurs due to high blood pressure and it is the cardinal feature in patients with heart muscle disease (cardiomyopathy), where it is also usually associated with body swelling of prominent engorged neck veins and enlarged liver. Heart attack and angina may also result in breathing difficulty at rest or during exertion. There are potent drugs that relieve circulatory congestion by bringing out extra fluid through urination (diuretics), augmentation of heart action (digitalis), unloading the burden on heart by their action on peripheral vasculature (nitrates, calcium channel blockers and ACE inhibitors). Definitive management includes ballooning of narrowed valves, and repair or replacement of grossly deformed heart valves. Shortening the dimensions of expanded left ventricle due to heart muscle disease by surgery (volume, reduction surgery) and cardiac transplant in patients with end stage heart failure are the other management strategies for very sick cardiac patients where breathlessness is the major symptom. Lung disease and anemias are other major causes of breathlessness, needing specific management approach.

4. Fatigue

As a symptom of heart disease, fatigue is a manifestation of poor circulation of oxygenated blood to working muscles. It can occur due to any of the diseases as mentioned already and the management of fatigue will, therefore, depend upon taking due care of the disease responsible for it. Once again, non-cardiac causes of fatigue like anemia, hypothyroidism, loss of excess electrolytes, like sodium and potassium, and water due to hot weather or diarrhoeal diseases must be kept in mind in patients presenting with fatigue and lethargy as the sole symptoms.

Giddiness, and transitory loss of consciousness or blockouts (syncope) are two other symptoms of importance in the management of heart patients. Patients with heart blocks and severe narrowing of aortic valve may present to the physician with history of syncope or unconsciousness; the management for the former is implanting pacemaker, while for the narrowed aortic valve, the recommended treatment is either balloon valvoplasty or surgery.

The corrective and curative management of heart disease depends on the right diagnosis of the underlying defect. A careful listening to the patient's symptoms (unfortunately becoming rare these days), detailed physical examination and a few necessary investigations often help in arriving at the correct diagnosis.

After having serviced the engine and rectifying its defects, it is once again of immense importance to observe certain preventive measures to avoid recurrence of such problems.

Various Preventive Management Strategies for Heart Care

1) Avoiding the use of unnecessary medication, specially sedatives, stimulants, any new drugs, alcohol and smoking during early pregnancy. These measures will help to prevent some congenital heart diseases, like holes in the heart and defects that result in blue babies.

2) Adequate and early treatment of sore throat with antibiotics during childhood will prevent rheumatic fever which is the cause of deformed valves in later life. Curative treatment for these valvular defects is prohibitively expensive, and rheumatic heart disease unfortunately occurs among people in poor socio-economic status.

Once rheumatic fever and rheumatic heart disease have been diagnosed in a person, a periodic three-weekly long acting penicillin injection will help in preventing recurrence of the disease (secondary prophylaxis).

3) Preventive management against heart attacks and angina includes: (a) Avoiding smoking (b) Early detection and effective treatment of hypertension (c) Control and treatment of high blood cholesterol by diet and drugs (d) Doing regular physical exercise and (e) Avoiding mental stress: "Those who wish to protect their heart and its roots (coronary arteries) must avoid what causes mental affliction." (Charaka — 1000 B.C.)

4) Prevention of Hypertension: Avoiding excess salt, weight control, doing regular physical exercise, avoiding excess alcohol ingestion, and practice of mental relaxation through meditation, yoga and music help in primary prevention of high blood pressure (hypertension).

5) Diet rich in vegetables, fruits, nuts, fish and vitamins, specially vitamins E and C and folic acid, are helpful in prevention of atherosclerotic heart disease (heart attacks). Cholesterol comes only from diet of animal origin like meat, milk and dairy products. There is no cholesterol in foods from vegetables and of plant origin.

Although undernutrition is a major problem in many developing countries including India, yet overnutrition is responsible for many cases of heart attacks and hypertension. Periodic fasting instead of frequent feasting will, perhaps, therefore, be a sound preventive management strategy for the well-being and long life of heart, the unique, always-working engine of our body.

2
MIND AND HEART

In youth we learn; in age we understand.
— Marie Von Ebner — *Eschenbach*

Apart from heredity and genetic factors, the tripod which supports longevity has these three legs: *Nutrition, Physical Exercise and Mind*. It is from the East that the West has taken much on writing about the role of mind in health and disease and laid the foundation for psychosomatic medicine (psycho—mind, soma—physical body). Many of the modern texts on mind are the translations from the original Sanskrit scripts done by German and English scholars. It is difficult to define mind, but what I wish to describe is the effect that the various thought processes result in the human system when a person faces different stressful situations in life on one hand, and when he is at peace with himself and with his surroundings on the other hand. In fact, it is the emotions on which many of us have very little control, that set our behaviour pattern and also regulate the secretion of various hormones into our circulation, thus governing the functioning of our body.

Stress and emotions have two aspects—the physiological and the psychological aspects. Under a stressful situation, there is a rise in pulse rate, a rise in blood pressure and an increase in oxygen demand by the tissues, an increase in cardiac output and a decrease in renal and splanchnic blood flows. This is what happens under stressful situations. If that is so, then the situation opposite of that, i.e., mental relaxation, will be giving us the beneficial effects by control of heart rate, blood pressure and desired distribution of blood flow to various organ systems. If someone is under undue tension and also starts smoking and consuming excess alcohol, a situation commonly seen in the industrialised world, longevity in such a person is bound to be adversely affected by the summation effect of smoking, excess alcohol, a disturbed mind and invariably accompanying lack of exercise. One has to see as to WHY some people take to excess smoking and drinking, and not merely order them to stop these habits as they are harmful for health in general and heart in particular. The root cause of excessive smoking and drinking habit lies in not having a control at the mind level. Being told harshly by the spouse not to drink or smoke does not generally help. On the other hand, what helps is talking at length, in privacy and intimately about harmful effects that excess drinking and smoking have on the: (i) individual (ii) family members (iii) employment potential and (iv) society at large. The heart is not the master of ceremonies but a slave to the master called mind. It is through the state of mind that most of the functions are accomplished either directly or through the heart and other vital organs. Both the frequency and force of contraction of the heartbeat, blood pressure and regional blood flow to various organs are, to a great extent, governed by the psyche or mind and the emotional state of the individual. Listen to the following dialogue between the Heart and the Mind, as to the supremacy of one over the other:

The Heart said to the Mind:
"I am the master,
The power-house of life,
steering the bloodstream
to sustain your existence.
Directing its flow,
to nerve, tissue and flesh,
which structure and mansion
the human consciousness
over which you preside,
by my grace, power and efforts."
Cool, crafty Mind,
so strong and assured,
smiled his naughty smile,
both mocking and indulgent,
and replied to the Heart:
"Your claim of mastery
over the human psyche
is correct and admissible,
for you truly sustain life.
But you are a mere pump
whose flow of the life stream
is controlled by my cells,
of great magic and complexity,
in moods of elation and serenity,
which can destroy or cerebrate life.
You are surely a great performer,
and your role is crucial,
to the tempo, duration and quality of life,
you confirm to the life-force,
and exploit its energy,
to spend or to hoard,
while I plan and direct.

*If I am calm and serene,
wise and compassionate,
your power-house function
is smoothly performed.
In my anger and turmoil,
confusion and fear,
your nuts, bolts and valves
shake, crack and even break.
I must be serene and disciplined,
calm and tranquil,
in sleep, wakefulness and vigour,
to relax well and perform."
The Heart and the Mind spoke in unison,
singing the song of life:
"For the breath and feel of life,
its expressions and potentials
of joy and creation,
we belong to each other.
If the mind guides the heart
in peace hope and faith,
and the heart keeps bouncing
in wholesome physical feats,
life's tempo is great to live
and to create."
Together let us make
Doctor Wasir's two potent "drugs"
"Mind" and "Heart"
for the care of the heart
and the glory of the mind.*

—Prem Kirpal

(Excerpted from author's book,
Heart to Heart—A Holistic Approach to Heart Care).

Emotions

There are two types of emotions: the positive emotions and the negative emotions. It is the negative emotions which give rise to stress. Desires, anger, greed and attachment for worldly pleasures result in increase of: (a) heart rate (b) blood pressure (c) rate pressure product (heart rate x systolic pressure). It is this double product (rate pressure product), which is important for the oxygen requirement by the heart and hence, the patient suffers when harbouring negative emotions. On the other hand, positive emotions like "selfless service", "giving without expectations in return" and "may I help you" attitude, result in peace, tranquillity, equilibrium to self and the people around. Positive emotions keep the blood pressure and heart rate under desirable control and, therefore, protect the heart and cardiovascular system against the adverse effects that are produced with negative emotions.

State of mind is closely related to human well-being, aging process, longevity and occurrence of certain fatal events such as heart attacks and cancer. Happiness and depression are the reflections of one's state of mind. Weather, trees and flowers around us are the same but at times we enjoy them, and at other times, we are so indifferent to these gifts of nature. When in power, the politicians become young and more energetic but when out of power, they suddenly appear more aged, the shine of their skin is replaced by wrinkles! The same is true of the bureaucrats in powerful positions. It is an interesting observation to watch them around when in powerful positions and after retirement. Some of those who do not find good alternative positions soon after retirement, the aging process descends on them overnight, and occurrence of heart attacks is not uncommon around this period.

Another familiar example of shortening of lifespan due to stress and depression is the occurrence of death of the individual within a few months of the demise of one's spouse, a close long term associate or a loved one in the family or among close friends. One's knowledge, study and faith in religion, spiritual heritage and mental make-up are helpful to withstand successfully the transition of retirement during the *vanaprastha ashram* in one's life.

Mental Relaxation

There are various ways by which one can achieve mental relaxation, and the most important ones practised in our country and abroad are the *Padmasana, Siddhasana* and *Shavasana*.

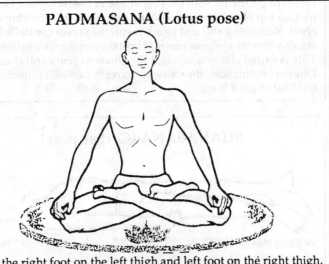

PADMASANA (Lotus pose)

Place the right foot on the left thigh and left foot on the right thigh, soles upwards, palms either on the knees or in the middle of groin facing upwards. Keeping the head erect and eyes closed, *Padmasana* is considered destroyer of Yogi's diseases.

Padmasana and *Siddhasana* are used during meditation and *Pranayaam* (breathing exercise), while *Shavasana* is the posture for achieving relaxation after doing most of the other *asanas* and at the end of the day.

SIDDHASANA (Adept's pose)

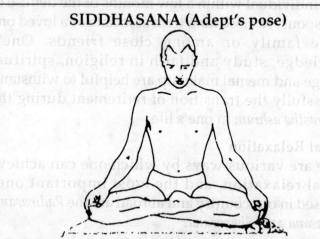

Press the perineum with the heel of one of the feet, place the other foot on top of the genitals. Having done this, rest the chin on the chest. Remaining still and steady, with the senses controlled, gaze steadily into the eyebrow centre; it breaks open the door to liberation. This is called *siddhasana*, ideal for Dharana (concentration) and Dhyana (meditation), the stairways to reach Samadhi (illumination), the final stage of Yoga.

SHAVASANA (Corpse pose)

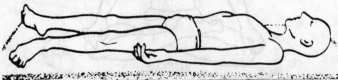

Lying flat on the ground with the face upwards, in the manner of a dead body, is *shavasana*. It removes tiredness and enables the mind and whole body to relax.

Normally, *Shavasana* is recommended for 15 to 20 minutes, but even if you try it for 5 to 10 minutes, specially in the evenings when you come back after a day's hard work, you will experience the relaxation which you will get by doing this *asana*. You just cannot get this physical and mental relaxation from any tranquilliser as you will get from the practice of *Shavasana*.

In the modern rat race, what is happening is that most of us cannot get even 20 minutes to half an hour for the type of *asanas* which I have mentioned. So what is the alternative? Here Lord Ganesha comes to our help—Lord Ganesha's posture, the way He sits, gave me the idea of *Ganeshasana* for the ever busy executives and physicians. During the day-to-day work, when you are working, in between your meetings or during a break, after seeing ten to fifteen patients, we can relax just three to five minutes in the *Ganeshasana* to practise *Yoganidra* (being awake yet we are detached from our usual environment). Through *Ganeshasana*, short bursts of *Yoganidra* of 3-5 minutes, one can get the desired mental relaxation. *Ganeshasana* can be practised in your work chair and in your formal dress during office hours.

The positive role of mind in prevention of heart attacks was very nicely summed up in *Charaka Samhita*: "The person desiring to protect from the adverse effects upon his heart, its roots (coronary blood vessels) and the contents therein should scrupulously avoid all that causes affliction of mind."

GANESHASANA

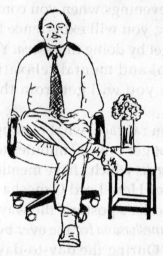

Ganeshasana is suitable for Yoganidra of short durations for mental relaxation during daily activities.

The modern cardiologists and the physicians tell you the same story in different ways and through slides and cassettes. Whatever gives you mental affliction should be avoided by modifying your reactions to the stressful situation in a positive way, in order to protect your heart from the harmful effects of stress and tension. Regarding the role of mind on heart, William Harvey in his treatise, *De Motus Cordis*, in 1628, mentions: "Every affliction of the mind that is attended with either pain or pleasure, hope or fear is the cause of an agitation whose influence extends to the heart."

Stress and Longevity
It is difficult to precisely define stress, but as a physician, I feel stress may be described as, "a

situation resulting from imbalance between one's environmental demands and the individual's capability to meet these demands."

And human response to stress can fall under three categories:

1) Effort without distress
2) Effort with distress
3) Distress without effort or (positive) effect.

Challenging and interesting stress is productive and beneficial, but when associated with fear and uncertainty, it becomes harmful as there is a perceived loss of control over the situation and its outcome. This type of stress is associated with increased neurohumoral activity (activity related to the nervous system and the endocrine system of the body) that proves harmful for the cardiovascular system by causing hypertension, angina, heart attacks, arrythmias and even sudden cardiac death.

3
LIFESTYLE AND LONGEVITY

O wherefore our age be revealing?
  Leave that to the registry books!
A man is as old as he's feeling
  A woman as old as she looks.

— MORTIMER COLLINS, *How Old Are You?*

Since the genesis of human race, there always have been endless efforts to find ways and means to prolong life and live longer. The royal physicians worked hard, and travelled far and wide in search of the magic herbs and precious metals that could enhance potency and prolong life. The ancient Indian system and science of medicine called *Ayurveda* itself originates from the concept of longevity (*ayu*—age/life, *veda or vidya*—knowledge) and the first few chapters of *Charaka Samhita* are devoted to longevity. While in earlier ages like *Satya Yuga*, *Treta* and *Dwapra* the human lifespan was 400, 300 and 200 years respectively, in the present *Kaliyug* it is of 100 years; approximately divided into four *ashrams* of 25 years each; starting with *brahamcharya*, going through *grhastha*, *vanprastha* and finally the *sanyas ashram*. The biblical lifespan, however, was of 70 years, i.e., three scores plus ten.

Eradication and control of many communicable diseases through the marvels of modern medicine, improved nutritional standards, advances in diagnostic technology, therapeutic interventions with many efficacious drugs, ballooning angioplasty, laser, stents, bypass operations and organ transplant surgery have greatly contributed to increase in the average lifespan of most nations.

The subject of longevity or living longer, therefore, is of great historical interest and of concern to every individual, physicians as well as non-physicians, for it deals with the extension of lifespan. Death is inevitable, yet everyone wants to defy it and live longer and longer and some may even be praying for immortality. No panacea or *sanjivini* has yet been invented for longevity. Living habits to a great extent have a bearing relationship with longevity.

The story of the relationship between the living styles and longevity is a long voyage from childhood to the elderly. The texts of *Charaka Samhita* and *Ayurveda* have dealt with the subject of aging (*ayur*) at great length. And how do we achieve it? Putting in the words as articulated in our *shastras*, it is a story moving from *balashram* to *sanyas ashram* through *grhastha ashram* and *vanprastha ashram*. That is how the story of longevity goes, whatever molecular medicine we may talk, when it comes to health care in general and prevention or control of the common diseases of present age such as coronary disease, hypertension, diabetes, obesity, osteoarthritis, cancer or AIDS, it comes down to the basic living habits, i.e., eating patterns (*aahaar*), smoking and drinking habits and our conduct (*aachaar*), thought processes (*vichaar*) and interpersonal social interactions (*vyvahaar*).

Problems Related to Lifestyle

Let us look at the various ailments related to lifestyle. Most of the present day killers and modern diseases which afflict the human being are related to the way of living and approach to life. Several psychosomatic disorders, and disorders like coronary disease, hypertension, obesity, diabetes, diet-related problems and lung cancer are all related directly or indirectly to lifestyles. The most dreadful disease of the present time is AIDS which is also related to one's lifestyle. If we care to probe deeper and trace roots of more modern killer diseases, I am sure, we can achieve longer life by mere modification in our living and eating habits.

Our living habits, including eating pattern, drinking and smoking habits, socio-economic factors and psycho-social factors, all these comprise what we term as "Lifestyle". This concept of lifestyle is obviously not a new phenomenon of this century. When we look into the past, we find that the father of medicine, Hippocrates, had mentioned about lifestyle several centuries back. While addressing the physicians, he had said: "If you wish to study medicine properly, in the first place, consider the seasons of the year, the waters, the ground and the mode in which the inhabitants live and what are their pursuits, whether they are fond of over-eating and over-drinking and given to sedentary living or are they fond of exercise and labour." The role of lifestyle to human well-being was thus well understood in the ancient era. We have from our own country, Guru Nanak, who compared the air to a teacher; the water to father; the earth, as the mother; and he said, it is the interaction of these through the days and nights that the whole universe continues. He said, *"Pawan guru, paani pita mataa dharat muhatt; divis raat doi dai daia khele sagal jagat."*

If you want to sum up the relationship of lifestyle to disease and you have on this list obesity, diabetes, hypertension, infections, AIDS, angina, accidents, ulcers, osteoarthritis, gallstones and lung disease, all these can be correlated to lifestyle. To put it simply, the cause of the various lifestyle-related diseases starting with "S": excessive *salt* intake, excessive *sugar* consumption, alcohol *(spirit)* abuse, *smoking, sedentary* lifestyle-related *stress* and inclusion of abnormal *sexual* behaviour will account for the AIDS. All these diseases are lifestyle-related disorders and potentially preventable.

Diet and Longevity

"In earlier times starvation consigned languishing bodies to death, now on the other hand, prosperity plunges them into the grave." — *Lucretius*

It is both under-eating and overeating which have been the problems affecting human longevity. Hence, moderation is the keyword for longevity. Starvation and famines used to kill large populations in the past, in the modern era it is overeating that takes away many precious lives through atherosclerotic heart disease, hypertension and stroke.

If you look at the modern diseases such as heart disease, high blood pressure, cancer and environment-related problems, I am sure you will agree that we don't have to go too far to the electron microscopes for their control and prevention. It can be done largely by regulating, modifying and monitoring the lifestyle of the human population, and a balanced diet has a major contribution in it.

Medical people normally talk of risk factors. Let us look from another angle. What are the protective factors or the factors which promote health and increase longevity? It is a view from a different angle and it is better to look at life from the positive side rather than all the time talking of factors for disease and sickness. Let us talk of the factors which promote health and increase longevity: Regular physical exercise, mental relaxation, avoiding smoking and consuming a diet rich in fibre, complex carbohydrates low in fats and refined carbohydrates. It is the diet we eat that I am going to discuss in the text that follows under the various sub-headings.

The most important thing is our nutrition *(aahaar)* on which we live. And when we talk of nutrition-related longevity, I will take you back to some solid data which has been collected by the World Health Organisation.

Over the centuries, as the industrialisation of the nations has occurred, an old system practised in our country of periodic, fasting or *vrat* which was a very common feature, has gradually given place to frequent *feasting*. There are now more frequent eating parties, sometimes even on weekdays. In this era of more eating, there is much less time being spent on physical exercise with the emerging of new living styles. And that in fact is the crux of the whole matter which results in various modern maladies as the intake of calorie increases and the output diminishes due to lack of exercise. The situation is often complicated by smoking and heavy alcohol ingestion.

The role of diet has been stressed very much in our ancient literature and it says thus: "Overeating, heavy and fatty meals, worries, sedentary habits and over-indulgence in sleep are the causes of several heart problems." (Charaka—1000 B.C.)

The pundits of modern medicine stress the same regarding heart ailments. It is not only the diet which you take but the environment in which you eat, that makes all the differences and that is why it was mentioned in Ayurveda: "Even the wholesome food taken in proper quantity does not get digested well due to anxiety, vigil, fear and anger" *(Charaka)*. Hence, it is at the dining table where you make or mar your health, prevent or promote health disorders.

If we keep these things in mind, I am sure we can prevent several diseases for which we have to unnecessarily spend lakhs of rupees. Coming to cardiac patients, balloon angioplasty is not generally less than a lakh of rupees and about 1/3 of these patients come back in course of a few months with recurrence of the same problem. Even for patients undergoing bypass heart surgery or CABG (Coronary Artery Bypass Graft) surgery, a lot of money is needed for such an operation (minimum of over one lakh rupees). Similarly, for the valve replacement operations, one heart valve operation costs about one lakh of rupees, and then the patient has to continue taking drugs lifelong, some drugs having a potential risk of bleeding if given in excess, and clotting of the valve will occur if the patient is undertreated with such drugs. Treatment for the clotted heart valve is again very expensive, at times the valve may have to be replaced with a new one. This disease unfortunately occurs in poor people. Whether it is the coronary heart disease treatment with angioplasty or bypass surgery, replacement of joints, heart valves, kidney, liver or the heart transplant, or the chemotherapy and radiotherapy for cancer, all these are prohibitively costly procedures both for the family and for the state, specially in the developing countries with meagre resources.

Obesity, Nutrition and Longevity

Obesity has a direct relation with disease, disability and death. Central obesity, i.e., waist bigger than hips (waist/hip ratio of one or above) is a risk factor for heart attacks. Except for some rare instance where an obese individual may enjoy good health into old age, generally, obesity is inversely proportional to long life as is evident from the life insurance data and population surveys. As the weight goes up so does the overall mortality in the various population (WHO). A Body Mass Index (BMI = wt. in kg. /ht. in metre^2) of above 25 is obesity. Here it is important to know that while computing BMI we divide a person's weight by square of his/her height in metre. For example, a person with a weight of 55 kg and height of 1.62 metres will have a BMI = 55 kg/1.62 x 1.62 metre^2 = 21.25, which is below 25, i.e., the person is not obese.

As the weight goes high, the cholesterol also goes high, and this equation is by and large diet-related. The good cholesterol called the HDL (High Density Lipoprotein), or the friendly cholesterol comes down as the body weight goes up. If that is so, then we know that we should eat things that do not increase cholesterol and lower HDL, as we know HDL is a protective factor against heart attacks. The dietary source of cholesterol is the food of animal origin such as milk, dairy products and meats.

The total body fat consumption and the cardio-vascular mortality is linearly correlated and the same is true with cholesterol levels. The cumulated data of various studies from several countries show that as the

Lifestyle and Longevity

cholesterol levels increase, so do the trends of mortality from cardio-vascular disease. And if we add smoking to obesity, then it adds fuel to the fire, thus further increasing mortality and morbidity, especially due to cardio-vascular disease in both males and females.

We have enough evidence that overweight shortens lifespan, and overweight by and large is the result of overeating and eating calorie-rich foods such as sweets and fried items. We must, therefore, attack the problem at its roots by restricting food intake to avoid becoming fat rather than going to various high cost slim centres, where again the results of weight control will only be temporary if the eating pattern is not changed to consume low calorie, high vitamin balanced protein diet and supplemented with regular physical exercise.

An American physician named Dean Ornish has written a book on reversal of atherosclerosis. He says that if you change your diet from non-vegetarian to vegetarian and you do regular physical exercise, practise yoga and meditation, you can reverse atherosclerosis, i.e., decrease the narrowing of your already partially blocked arteries. And he learnt all this during one of his meetings with a yogi from India. Back home in America he did some study by changing the living habits or the lifestyles of a group of people and showed that you can actually regress atherosclerosis by what I would call *Food for Heart*, a concept that has been detailed in my earlier book *Traditional Wisdom and Heart Care*. Food for heart comprises: (1) A balanced diet containing high fibre, complex carbohydrates like tubers, roots (2) Regular physical exercise and (3) Relaxed mind. This is the *tripod of longevity*. It should be clearly understood that while taking a vegetarian diet does not give permanent immunity from heart attacks, consuming meat in moderation, specially white meat and fish, along with the usual quota of vegetables and fruits may not be harmful for health in general and the heart in particular. If uric acid and blood cholesterol levels are normal the mixed non-vegetarian and vegetarian diet (omnivorous habit) is better for a healthy heart.

It is a common saying that we become what we eat, and another one saying that we should eat to live and not live to eat. In fact, I strongly believe that the arena where you make or mar your health is the dining table, not only the food on it but it is the environment during eating that affects our health and longevity. Food that protects against heart attacks, high blood pressure stroke and cancer, the main modern killers, should be a balanced diet comprising vegetables, whole fruits, coarse grains, coarse ground flour bread and not the one made from refined flour *(maida)*, milk and curd in moderation and avoiding extra salt and excess alcohol consumption. Diets rich in potassium (fresh whole fruits, vegetables, nuts) and low in sodium (avoiding preserved foods and pickles) are helpful in prevention of hypertension and stroke. The reason why there is a high prevalence of high blood pressure, heart attacks and stroke in the urban populations and industrialised nations is that their diet habits have changed to consume the fast foods containing large amounts of salt, preservatives, fats and less of protective elements like potassium, vitamins and fibre. The damage is compounded by intake of excess alcohol, smoking and lack of physical exercise—which invariably go with the neo-rich affluent societies lacking knowledge on health and hygiene.

The ancient wisdom of Ayurveda was so impressed with the importance of diet *(aahaar)* to human well-being and longevity that the foods were accordingly divided into (a) *saatvik* (the supreme) — including vegetables, fruits, curd, honey etc. (b) *raajsik* (for physical vigour and vitality) — high protein foods (c) *taamsik* (inferior quality food) — highly spiced, salted and leftovers. When we look seriously into this matter, most of the major risk factors for heart attacks, hypertension and stroke, i.e., obesity, high blood cholesterol, smoking and lack of physical exercise are controllable through our own efforts and by modifying our lifestyle.

Paul Dudly White, the noted cardiologist from America had said: "Heart disease before the age of 80 is not God's will but due to our own faults." I think it was a very strong message, he sent across to all of us who deal with the prevention of cardiovascular problems by regulation of lifestyle. Dr. Paul White practised what he preached about the role of lifestyle in promoting positive health. He did live much beyond the age of three scores plus ten.

4
DIET, ALCOHOL, SMOKING AND EXERCISE

While one finds company in himself and his pursuits, he cannot feel old, no matter what his years may be.

— AMOS BRONSON ALCOTT

Diet in Prevention of Heart Attacks

Cardiovascular diseases and cancer account for the maximum number of deaths and disability in adults all over the world. Some decades ago, this situation existed only in advanced countries but the developing countries now appear to be catching up fast. The print and visual media have a role in the fast changes that have occurred in people's living habits, including their dietary habits.

Although undernutrition may be a problem for millions of those below the poverty line, a large part of the population, specially the urban inhabitants, suffer from overnutrition. The adverse effects of the "affluent" diet characterised by excess calorie foods rich in fats, refined sugars and sodium, but deficient in complex carbohydrate (source of dietary fibre) and potassium have resulted in high incidence of coronary heart disease, hypertension and cerebrovascular disease (strokes).

Alcohol, an accepted dietary component (when used in small amounts) has been responsible for causing hypertension and heart muscle disease (cardiomyopathy) when used in excess. Other diseases which result from "affluent" diets include: diabetes, gallstones, obesity, osteoarthritis, dental caries and certain intestinal disorders. The major risk factor for stroke (brain attacks) is hypertension where excess salt intake, alcohol and obesity play a major role, all related to faulty diet habits. Through changes in eating habits, avoiding fats, refined sugars and lowering alcohol and salt consumption, several developed nations, like the US and Australia, have been able to drastically lower the incidence of heart attacks, stroke and hypertension. This has led to worldwide interest in socio-political acceptance of the urgent need for prevention-oriented national health policies on the incidence of diet-related cardiovascular diseases such as coronary artery disease, hypertension and stroke.

The common cardiovascular disorders that come under the diet-disease relationship are: atherosclerotic coronary, cerebral, renal, splanchnic, and peripheral artery diseases. Among the blood lipids, it is specially the Low Density Lipoprotein (LDL), Triglycerides, Very Low Density Lipoprotein (VLDL) and Lipoprotein (a) {Lp(a)} which are some of the lipids that have been incriminated in the causation and aggravation of atherosclerotic plaques (fatty streaks). HDL (High Density Lipoprotein), on the other hand, has a preventive effect against atherosclerosis. During the Second World War, people in countries like Norway, where the fat consumption decreased markedly, suffered less heart attacks. Atherosclerosis has been found to regress during starvation.

Coronary heart disease due to narrowing of blood vessels as a result of atherosclerosis is the main cause of mortality and morbidity in most developed countries. The exact cause of atherosclerosis is not known but from the environmental observation and epidemological studies in the transmigration populations (Indians in UK and Japanese in USA), changes in the lifestyles including changes in eating habits have been found to play a major role through alterations in blood lipids and impaired glucose-insulin relationship. The role of cholesterol in causing atherosclerosis has now been well established by several experimental, clinical and epidemological studies. A strong correlation has also been seen between

The relationship between saturated fat intake and incidence of death from coronary heart disease in males in seven countries over a ten-year period

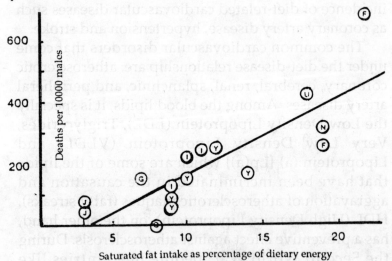

Saturated fat intake as percentage of dietary energy

Note. F = Finland, G = Greece, I = Italy, J = Japan, N = Netherlands, U = United States, Y = Yugoslavia. The extremes in intake often apply to non-European populations.

(WHO TRS 797)

the intake of saturated fats and serum cholesterol. This forms a strong case for prevention of coronary heart disease through diet control and lowering the intake of fatty foods and cholesterol-rich diet. It is worth noting here that the dietary sources of exogenous cholesterol are of animal origin-like meat, milk and dairy products. Foods from the vegetable kingdom—all vegetables, fruits, fresh or dry fruits — do not contain cholesterol.

Populations with low average cholesterol levels like rural China (125 mg per cent) and Japan (165 mg per cent) have very low incidence of coronary heart disease compared to countries where cholesterol levels are high, such as Finland (270 mg per cent). In a multi-country study, populations with serum cholesterol level below 200 mg per cent had average saturated fat intakes between 3-10 per cent and low mortality from coronary heart disease. In populations with saturated fat intake of above 10 per cent, a progressive increase in coronary mortality was recorded.

The different mono- and poly-unsaturated fatty acids are said to have a protective role in coronary artery disease. The Mediterranean diet is rich in total fat intake (40 per cent) but a large part of it comes as mono-unsaturated fatty acids (olive oil) and these populations have a low incidence of coronary heart disease. Eskimos consume large amounts of total fat but as it comes from n-3 poly-unsaturated fatty acids, mainly from the fish, they have low incidence of coronary artery disease.

Out of the three major risk factors for coronary heart disease, viz., hypertension, high blood cholesterol and smoking, two are definitely related to diet and all three are related to lifestyle. It has also been shown in several studies that vegetarians have low serum cholesterol levels than meat-eaters, and so the incidence of coronary heart disease is also lower in vegetarians. Reduction in serum cholesterol levels, either by diet or drugs, has resulted in lowering the incidence of coronary artery disease. For primary prevention of coronary heart disease (heart attacks), it is thus mandatory that the serum cholesterol levels should be kept low, preferably below 200 mg per cent and LDL below 100 mg %.

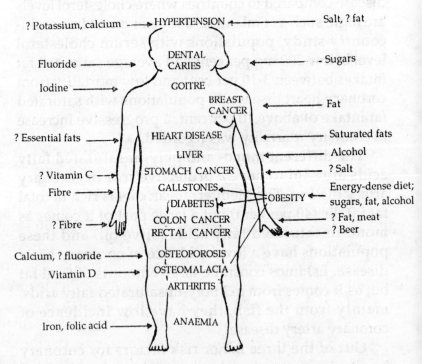

Diet-related Health Problems
Source: WHO Regional Publications, European Series No. 24

To achieve this the total fat consumption should be reduced to 30 per cent of total calorie intake, different unsaturated fatty acids to contribute up to 20 per cent of energy, and the cholesterol content of diet should not exceed 300 mg/day. Dietary fibre, found in coarse complex carbohydrates like tubers, roots, legumes from the vegetable kingdom, also help in keeping the serum cholesterol low.

Hypertension is closely related both to heart attacks and brain attacks (strokes). The cause of high blood pressure in adults is unknown in over 90 per cent of cases. There are, however, certain factors which, when present, tend to increase blood pressure. These factors include: being overweight, physical inactivity (sedentary lifestyle), excess salt intake and alcohol intake of more than two ounces equivalent of whisky per day. Hostile environment and mental tension causing constriction of arterioles, increased heart rate and cardiac output, are the other factors which raise blood pressure. Diet and living habits thus contribute largely to the genesis and aggravation of blood pressure and through this to higher incidence of myocardial infarction (heart attacks) and cerebrovascular disease (stroke). A salt intake of less than 6 gm daily, vegetarian diet rich in potassium and a decrease in total calories are, therefore, the dietary measures to control and prevent high blood pressure which will also help to lower the overall incidence of cardiovascular and cerebrovascular diseases.

Use of drugs to lower blood pressure have resulted in significant reduction in stroke incidence, but the fall in coronary disease has not been that impressive. This is because many drugs, in order to lower blood pressure (thiazides, betablockers), increase serum cholesterol, thus tilting the balance against lowering coronary disease. With the use of safe drugs that do not raise the serum cholesterol, effective antihypertensive treatment in future will help in preventing both coronary and cerebrovascular disease.

Learning from the experience of some developed countries which already have faced and managed the problem of cardiovascular disease by dietary interventions and changes in lifestyle, other nations must incorporate adequate dietary plans in their national health policies as preventive strategies for cardiovascular disease.

Curative treatment for heart disease, like ballooning or bypass is very expensive and beyond the reach of many individuals and even governments. Recurrence of the disease even after bypass surgery or angioplasty is not uncommon. On the current assumptions, cardiovascular disease will emerge as a substantial public health problem in practically every country by the end of this century. Opening more hospitals and bypass centres will not really solve the problem of cardiovascular disease. Primary prevention is the answer if we have to usher in the 21st century as healthy nations.

Many premature deaths and disability due to cardiovascular diseases are preventable through modification of dietary habits and other lifestyles. In view of the prohibitive costs incurred in the curative treatment of cardiovascular diseases (angioplasty, laser, stents, atherectomy, valve replacements, bypass surgery and heart transplant operations) and the expensive care in the so-called intensive care units, primary prevention through lifestyle changes is not only a medical and social responsibility but an economic necessity.

Whatever may be the risk factor a prudent diet can prevent/delay the progression of heart disease. *(See figure on the following page)*

INTERRELATIONSHIPS BETWEEN DIET AND OTHER RISK FACTORS

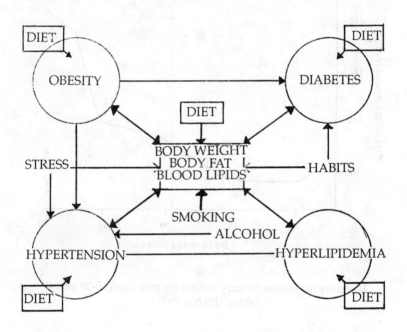

Modified from *Diet and Heart Disease* by Ghafoorunissa & K. Krishnaswamy.

Food Rich in Cholesterol

Meat and its products: Hen egg (yellow), liver, kidney, oysters, shrimp, crab, pork ribs, pork, lamb, mutton (goat).

Milk and its products: Ice-cream, butter, cream, animal fat.

FATNESS AND FITNESS DON'T GO TOGETHER

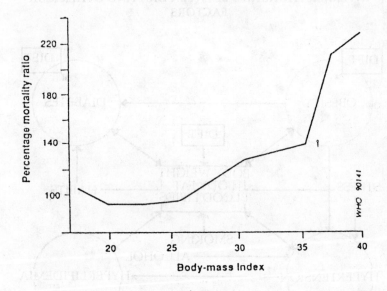

Mortality in relation to body weight for men aged 15-39 years
(Who TRS No. 797)

Food with No Cholesterol
Cereals and pulses, vegetables, fruits, dry fruits, nuts.

High blood cholesterol should be controlled with diet modification and physical exercise. A very low cholesterol level is also not good for health, especially when achieved with the use of cholesterol lowering drugs. Certain levels of cholesterol are essential for efficient functioning of the nervous system and the synthesis of hormones, including sex hormones.

Cholesterol Content of Various Food Items*

Food	Quantity (g)	Household measure	Cholesterol content (mg)
Meat & Its Products			
Yellow of eggs	100 g	Two	420 mg
Chicken (broiler)	100 g	1 portion	60 mg
Mutton (goat) (medium fat/lean)	100 g	3-4 pieces	65 mg
Liver	100 g	4-6 pieces	300 mg
Kidney	100 g	2 pieces	150 mg
Brain	100 g	7 tbsps	250 mg
Pork	100 g	1 slice	70 mg
Oysters	100 g	1 portion	230-470 mg
Shrimp	100 g	1 portion	150 mg
Crab	100 g	1 portion	145 mg
Pork ribs	100 g	Two	105 mg
Lamb	100 g	1 portion	70 mg
Milk & Its Products			
Whole milk	100 ml	1 small cup	11 mg
Skimmed milk	100 ml	1 small cup	2.4 mg
Cream	100 ml	1 small cup	100 mg
Butter	100 g	1 small cup	240 mg
Cheese	100 g	4 slices	16 mg
Plain ice-cream	100 g	1 small cup	375 mg
Animal fat	100 g	1 small cup	90 mg

* Source: *Nutritive Value of Indian Foods*, National Institute of Nutrition, Hyderabad, 1990.

Food items recommended for patients with high blood pressure or those with heart disease.

Potassium and Sodium in Dietary Items

High on Potassium*		Low on Sodium*	
Name of Food Items	Potassium (mg/100 g)	Name of Food Items	Sodium (mg/100 g)
Bengal gram	808 mg	Bajra	8 mg
Chana	720 mg	Rice flakes	12 mg
Black gram	800 mg	Vermicelli	8 mg
Lobia	1132 mg	Maida	8 mg
Green gram (whole)	844 mg	Onion (small)	4 mg
Moth	1096 mg	Potato	6 mg
Green gram (split)	1160 mg	Sweet potato	4 mg
Red gram	1104 mg	Yam	4 mg
Peas, dry	724 mg	Green gourd	2 mg
Spinach	206 mg	Brinjal	3 mg
Arbi	280 mg	French beans	4 mg
Sweet potato	500 mg	Lady'sfingers	7 mg
Apricots, fresh	430 mg	Peas	8 mg
Sweet lime	490 mg	Pumpkin	6 mg
Peaches	453 mg	Gooseberry	4 mg
Plums	247 mg	Guava	5 mg
Phalsa	351 mg	Orange	5 mg
Buffalo milk	140 mg	Papaya, ripe	6 mg
Curd	260 mg	Peaches	2 mg
		Phalsa	4 mg

* *Source: Nutritive Value of Indian Foods*, National Institute of Nutrition, Hyderabad, 1990.

Alcohol

Unlike the habit of smoking that came to India about 500 years ago, use of alcohol possibly dates back to times immemorial, as its descriptions are available in the ancient texts both in India and abroad. According to the Ayurvedic text *Charaka Samhita: Wine, if taken properly, gives pleasant intoxication and produces exhilaration, energy, contentment, freedom from disorders, sexual potency and strength.* This description surpasses most of the modern texts of the beneficial effect of mild to moderate alcohol consumption, taken properly. It is also well known to us from several epidemiological studies the world over, that heart attacks are less common in those populations that consume moderate amounts of alcohol. Wine consumption (fermented alcohol) is perhaps more cardioprotective than the distilled alcohol as appears from the French observation of less coronary disease compared to the neighbouring UK and other countries where whisky consumption is more prevalent. Excessive alcohol consumption (more than two ounces per day), however, results in major medical, social and economic problems, for the individual, their families and for the state. The medical problems include: (i) dependence (addiction) (ii) liver cirrhosis (iii) cognitive and neurological disorders (iv) accidents (v) hypertension (vi) arrhythmias (vii) heart muscle disease (cardiomyopathy) (viii) foetal defects in mothers who drink alcohol (ix) stroke and (x) increased overall mortality.

The harmful social and economic impact of excessive alcohol consumption is also well recognised by every country. The WHO has recognised that the problems related to excessive alcohol intake rank among the world's major health problems, constituting serious hazards for human health, welfare and life. Although a small amount of alcohol consumption may be beneficial for prevention of coronary artery disease and improving social interaction yet the harmful effects, medical, social and economic of alcohol abuse, clearly outweigh its cardioprotective effects. It has been estimated that the overall costs of alcohol misuse such as from health-related disorders, social problems, accidents and due to divorces and imprisonment are greater than from smoking and use of illicit drugs. If individuals could limit alcohol intake to safe levels (up to two drinks per day), then it may be considered as a tonic for improving the quality of life and possibly longevity too by preventing coronary heart disease. But excessive alcohol use results in increased disability and death thus diminishing the quality of life and longevity. "Safe drinking" is like "safe sex", it brings pleasure and enjoyment, while excessive drinking brings more disease and deaths like "unsafe sex". The outcome of excessive alcohol intake is beautifully described in the Ayurvedic texts: *When overpowered by wine, happiness and enjoyment disappear, mental aberrations arise, culminating in unconsciousness and death (Charaka Samhita).*

Smoking

Smoking habit decreases longevity and the decrease in lifespan is directly proportionate to the number of cigarettes smoked per day. Apart from the shortening of number of years that a smoker lives, the quality of living during these years is adversely affected by the occurrence of diseases like bronchitis, angina, hoarseness of voice, decrease in sexual potency and suffering from claudication pain of the legs. Tobacco consumption is a major cause of death and disability both in the developed and developing countries—more so now in the latter.

Not only does the smoking habit adversely affect the smoker, but those who happen to be near the smoker also bear its brunt. The smoker, at least, may at times be enjoying and feeling relaxed during the act, but those around him suffer as passive smokers by inhailing "second hand" smoke and undergoing the discomfort of being in the vicinity of the smoker. The exact magnitude of disease and disability due to passive smoking may be difficult to gauge, but many innocent souls suffer for no fault of theirs! Moving a step ahead of passive smoking, the habit of smoking during pregnancy results in low birth weight of the yet-to-be-born, premature births and spontaneous abortions.

The relationship of smoking to problems related to health is so strong that from time to time the World Health Organisation (WHO) has been coming out with topical issues in its periodicals focusing on the tobacco menace. On April 7 every year, 'WHO Day', many anti-smoking campaigns have been launched for public awareness against the habit of smoking. Meanwhile, May 31 each year is observed as 'No Tobacco Day'.

The list of the diseases that result from tobacco consumption is a rather lengthy one and includes:
a) Lung diseases, like bronchitis and lung cancer.
b) Heart diseases like heart attacks and sudden death.

c) Diseases of blood vessels—like hardening of arteries that result in a diminished blood supply to the limbs causing pain in legs on walking (claudication).
d) Cancer of oral cavity (like tongue and mouth), voice-box and urinary bladder.
e) Defects in the foetus and newborn babies of smoking mothers.
f) Impotence and impaired libido due to atherosclerosis of blood vessels to genitalia.

Each year about 3 million people die in the world due to tobacco-related diseases, amounting to one death every 10 seconds due to smoking. (1) In India, about 8 lakh persons die each year due to their tobacco consumption habit, i.e., 2,200 persons die every day due to tobacco-related diseases including cancer of various organs such as lung, voice-box, mouth, urinary bladder and uterus. If tobacco consumption is not controlled, then in the year 2000, there will be 2.5 lakh persons in India with cancer due to tobacco. India has the highest number of cancer of oral cavity because of the common habit of tobacco chewing. Tobacco came to India as far back as 1558 and its harmful effects became evident in the seventeenth century. A clear link of smoking with lung cancer was established by 1950. The production of cigarettes has been rising in India by about one per cent annually and that of *bidis* by about 5 per cent per year. The mean Indian consumption of cigarettes per year is about 200 per adult plus approximately 300 gms of *bidis*. (2) *Bidis* are not any safer than cigarettes. The tar and nicotine content of *bidi* is higher than that in the cigarettes, though the tobacco content maybe 1/4 of the cigarettes. Unlike in the developed countries where the tobacco consumption has fallen in the last few decades, in developing countries including India, consumption of tobacco continues to rise.

Smoking and Heart Disease

Smoking is a major contributors towards deaths and disability from cardiovascular disease. Smokers have 3 to 4 times greater risk of developing a heart attack. In India, out of the 60 lakh persons getting heart attack annually, 13 lakh are due to smoking. Smoking is not only one of the three major risk factors for heart attacks (the others being hypertension and high-blood lipids), but it can also cause a heart attack early. In a study of myocardial infarction (heart attacks) in the young (less than 40 years age) conducted at the department of cardiology of the All India Institute of Medical Sciences, it was found that the only risk factor in majority of the patients was cigarette smoking. How does smoking result in this havoc? By one or more of the following ways:

i) By causing acute narrowing (spasm) of coronary arteries that supply oxygenated blood to heart muscle. This may result in acute heart attack, angina, arrhythmias and sudden death.

ii) By increasing the adhesiveness or stickiness of the circulating blood platelets that may result in clot formation inside the arteries supplying the heart and brain, thus increasing the chances of heart attack and stroke among smokers.

iii) During smoking, the heart rate and blood pressure also rise, resulting in greater workload for the heart, which an already diseased heart may not stand well. This will result in heart failure.

iv) Aggravation of atherogenesis (narrowing) of arteries is another anatomical impairment. Apart from heart attack and sudden cardiac death, smoking is responsible for higher incidence of atherosclerotic disease (fatty deposits) of abdominal and femoral arteries, malignant hypertension, peripheral arterial disease and chronic corpulmonale, a disease still quite common in India and very much under control through avoidance of smoking in some other countries.

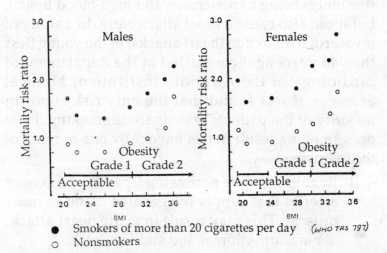

Smoking, body weight and risk of mortality (WHO - TRS 797)

The metabolic harmful effects of smoking include:
a) Increase in total cholesterol.
b) Increased triglycerides.
c) Decrease in HDL.

All these metabolic abnormalities are related to the process of atherogenesis that ultimately results in heart attacks and brain attacks (strokes). Even after bypass surgery the grafts get blocked early if patients do not quit smoking. The beneficial effect of various drugs, such as nitrates and betablockers, used in the treatment of heart diseases and hypertension is less marked in smokers compared to non-smokers. Malignant hypertension is more likely to occur in smokers.

Smoking and the use of contraceptive pills form an unholy alliance for increased mortality from heart attacks and stroke. Coronary heart disease incidence is higher in smoking women, but it affects more severely those who smoke and also use contraceptive pills.

Within about two years of quitting smoking, most of the risk ascribed to it seems to disappear except in heavy smokers where it may take longer. It is thus clear from the above stated facts, observations and the experience that smoking habit shortens lifespan. Cessation of smoking habit and global control on tobacco production by providing alternative crops for the farmers and suitable employment to those who are laid off their jobs from tobacco industry, will prove to be yet another step forward in increasing human longevity. Considering the overall huge expenditure on all the health problems related to smoking, the revenue returns from the tobacco industry may not be their worth. Health of the nations is perhaps, more important, than the wealth of the nations.

Physical Exercise in Heart Care

Alongwith a balanced diet, physical exercise has a major role in achieving long and healthy life. We know physically active populations have a higher longevity than the physically inactive or sedentary. The studies of the Harvard alumni have shown that the medical students when followed for twenty years who remained physically active, their longevity was better than those who remained physically sedentary. Once again I go back to our ancient wisdom of ayurveda which said: "The bodily movement which is meant for producing firmness and strength is known as physical exercise and it should be done in moderation." A recent study reported in the most widely circulated medical journal, *New England Journal of Medicine*, gave us some scientific data that strenuous physical exercise is harmful and as stated above we have a recorded mention of the same in our ancient texts about 25 centuries back. By physical exercise, it was stated in the ayurveda text of *Charaka Samhita: One gets lightness in the body, capacity to work, firmness, tolerance of difficulties, diminution of impurity and stimulation of metabolism.* This is what has been stated regarding the positive effects and promotive role of physical exercise in relation to longevity in our ancient texts on health. The modern research tells us that the beneficial effects of exercise are through: (1) increase in life of certain types of protein (2) decrease in hepatic lipase (3) decrease in insulin resistance (4) decrease in hyperinsulnemia (excessive insulin in blood) (5) decrease in cholesterol and triglycerides, LDL and VLDL and (6) increase in the friendly cholesterol HDL.

Physical exercise also normalises blood pressure in persons with mild hypertension. I did some work on this subject 25 years ago by putting young people with mild hypertension on a programme of physical exercise, bicycling on alternative days for an hour for a period of three months. We found that both systolic and diastolic pressure were lower than what they had started with. And there are other studies also showing that physically active professionals or in those with professions which involve more physical activity, the prevalence of hypertension is lower in such individuals than in those who are engaged in sedentary professions. This was also the observation made by us in a study on the prevalence of hypertension at All India Institute of Medical Sciences (AIIMS) campus done in the early eighties. In addition to the objective benefits mentioned above, physical exercise also gives you a feeling of well-being and helps you to avoid obesity which is one of the enemies of longevity. Those who are doing it, they become "addicts" to exercise, the day they cannot go for exercise, they feel unwell. That happens through secretion into the body of what we call endorphines, which are related to morphine-like substances. The best way to achieve mental and physical relaxation and to get a feeling of well-being is not through tranquillisers and sedatives or alcohol but it is through doing regular physical exercises. Those who do it know it and those who do not do it will know it only when they start doing physical exercises regularly.

Regular practice of dynamic (isotonic) exercise done in moderation, prevents diseases, promotes positive health and thus prolongs lifespan by:

(1) Control on body weight and avoiding obesity.
(2) Rate-pressure (pulse rate x systolic blood pressure) product is kept low in those who do regular physical exercise, and this helps in

economising on cardiac work and makes the heart live longer and healthier.

(3) Increase in exercise capacity and muscle power through training of muscles to extract more oxygen and work more efficiently at the given oxygen availability.

(4) There is an overall improvement in the body chemistry such as a fall in blood sugar levels, cholesterol, tryglyceroids LDL and an increase in the beneficial blood lipid HDL. The higher the HDL, the better it is to prevent heart attacks. Exercises help to achieve higher HDL levels. Persons with any ailments, specially, heart disease, should start an exercise programme only after consulting a physician, and must avoid isometric (static) exercise such as weightlifting, stretching and breath-holding exercises. (5) An overall feeling of well-being is a unique achievement coming through regular physical exercise. This combination of physical and mental relaxation achieved through physical exercise is unparalleled by any tonic or drug.

Physical exercise adds not only years to life but also life to years: Examples of isotonic (dynamic) exercises are: Brisk walking, swimming, rowing, and other outdoor games like tennis, golf and badminton. Walking is the best mode of doing regular exercise which requires no equipment, money, material or membership of a club!

5
BLOOD PRESSURE—HIGH AND LOW

> The riders in a race do not stop short when they reach the goal. There is a little finishing canter before coming to a standstill. There is time to hear the kind voice of friends and to say to one's self: "The work is done".
> — JUSTICE OLIVER WENDELL HOLMES, *Radio Address on his 90th birthday, 8 March, 1931*

There is a certain force which facilitates the maintaining of circulation of blood in our body and that force is termed as blood pressure. If this force is very high, beyond certain limits, a condition known as hypertension or high blood pressure, it will adversely affect the vital organs like brain, heart and kidneys resulting in stroke, heart attack, angina and kidney failure. In general, the life insurance companies' data show that the higher the pressures the lower the longevity. High blood pressure is a strong risk factor for longevity. On the other hand, if the blood pressure suddenly falls too low like in cases of dehydration due to severe diarrhoea, vomiting, heat exhaustion and high fevers, or due to extensive injury to body or heart muscle (massive heart attack), then also the whole body suffers due to lack of oxygenated blood supply to the vital organs, thereby resulting in cell damage and death if the blood pressure is not restored within reasonable time.

This brings us to the question — What is *normal* blood pressure? Before we define the level of normal blood pressure, it, would be relevant to mention here that blood pressure is encountered in two phases, i.e., an upper or *systolic* and the lower or *diastolic* pressure. The upper pressure corresponds to the phase of cardiac cycle during its contraction, i.e., *systole* and the lower pressure corresponds to the resting phase or *diastole*. A normal person does not have a fixed value of blood pressure. Unlike body temperature which is more or less fixed for the human beings in normalcy at 37°C (98.6°F), blood pressure reading varies from time to time, depending upon the physical and mental state of the individual and as per the needs of the body. During physical exercise as the heartbeat increases both in frequency and force of contraction the systolic blood pressure rises. In fact, if during physical exercise the systolic blood pressure does not rise above the individual's normal resting pressure, it is considered a sign of diseased heart.

Blood pressure varies with age. At the time of birth, the pressure normally is around 60-70/35-40 mm Hg and as a child grows, so does the blood pressure. And in adulthood, a reading of 120/80 mm Hg is considered as average normal. In most of the industrialised and urban populations of the world, there is an increase in both the systolic and diastolic pressure, more so, in the former with the advancing age. In women, the rise is steeper after their menopause. There are, however, some isolated tribal populations where the pressure has not been found to rise with aging. These tribes are characterised by: (1) living in isolation from the mainstream of civilised

Blood Pressure—High and Low

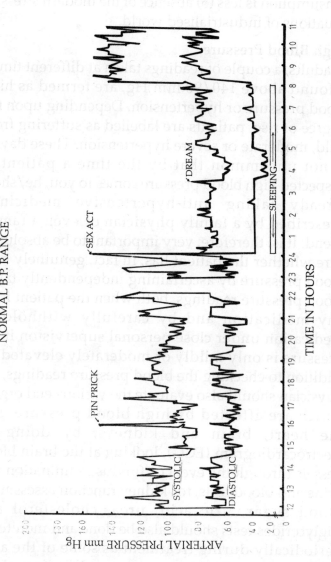

24 Hours Blood Pressure record

world (2) they are physically active (3) consume diets with excess of vegetables and fruits (4) salt consumption is less (5) absence of the modern stressful situations of industrialised world.

High Blood Pressure

In adults, a couple of readings taken at different times, if found above 140/90 mm Hg, are termed as high blood pressure or hypertension. Depending upon the degree of rise, patients are labelled as suffering from mild, moderate or severe hypertension. These days it is not uncommon that by the time a patient of suspected high blood pressure comes to you, he/she is already taking anti-hypertensive medicines, prescribed by a family physician or even a family friend. It is, therefore, very important to be absolutely sure whether the patient has, in fact, genuinely high blood pressure by ascertaining independently taken blood pressure readings, both when the patient is on any medication and by carefully withholding medication under close personal supervision if the pressure is only mildly or moderately elevated. In addition to checking the blood pressure readings, the physician should also evaluate the various end organs which are affected by high blood pressure, i.e., the heart, brain and kidneys, by doing an electrocardiogram (ECG), looking at the brain blood vessels through the eye, i.e., fundus examination and urine and blood tests, for kidney function assessment. Blood sugar, uric acid, urea, cholesterol and triglycerides tests should also be done and monitored periodically during treatment as some of the anti-hypertensive drugs may adversely affect these parameters.

Blood Pressure—High and Low

Symptoms
High blood pressure is, by and large, considered a silent disease, but I do not think it is that silent, as it has so far been believed to be. Heaviness in head, not simply a headache, pressure in the back of head, impaired vision, breathlessness on exertion, heaviness in whole body, lack of concentration in mental work, sleeplessness and increased irritability could be some of the pointers asking for a check-up of blood pressure and, therefore, should not be ignored. Marked palpitation, profuse sweating and headache, all these signs should make us suspect some of the curable conditions of hypertension. Similarly, weakness and fatigue or pain in legs on walking, or general weakness along with one or more of the above-mentioned symptoms should make one suspect and look for specific causes of high blood pressure called secondary hypertension.

Management
After a person is diagnosed to be having high blood pressure, an attempt should be made to look for any specific curable cause of hypertension like kidney disease, narrowing of upper segment of aorta or constriction of any of the major arteries, specially the renal arteries that supply pure blood to the kidneys. Once a specific cause is found by various investigations including sometimes angiography, ultrasonography, CT (Computerised Tomography) scan and even MRI (Magnetic Resonance Imaging), the cure for hypertension may be possible by either surgery or balloon angioplasty. Otherwise, in most of the cases of hypertension in adults, they have to be treated with drugs. Non-drug measures like:

(1) Weight control (2) Avoiding excess salt consumption (3) Avoiding alcohol (4) Doing regular physical exercise, and (5) Mental relaxation achieved through practice of meditation, music and yoga are often helpful in management of mild and moderate hypertension while for patients of severe hypertension, the drug requirement is reduced by practice of these non-pharmacological measures. Those who are taking anti-hypertensive drugs for a long time, must get their blood tests done periodically to check if any of the drugs is causing some adverse side-effects. They should also report to their physicians if any side-effects are noted, such as muscle weakness, cough and sexual difficulties as some anti-hypertensive drugs are likely to cause these side-effects in some individuals.

Low Blood Pressure

One does not normally like to label a person as suffering from *Low Blood Pressure*. There is no such disease as low blood pressure. If blood pressure is found exceptionally low, one should look for an underlying reason for that, like a silent heart attack, dehydration due to severe gastroenteritis, extreme fasting and unmonitored excess use of diuretics — the drugs that result in more urination. In hot and humid climates, there is often excessive water and electrolyte loss in sweating and this results in fall in blood pressure also. It is, therefore, advisable, that those working in such hot and humid surroundings must take adequate amount of fluid and salt to prevent occurrence of low blood pressure. The dose requirement of various anti-hypertensive drugs should also be reduced for the same reasons during the summer months.

6

ENVIRONMENTAL POLLUTION, HEART DISEASES AND LONGEVITY

Like a morning dream, life becomes more and more bright the longer we live, and the reason of everything appears more clear. What has puzzled us before seems less mysterious, and the crooked paths look straighter as we approach the end.

— JEAN PAUL RICHTER

Life thrives on two types of environment, the external environment from which the organism gets its food and air to survive, and the internal environment, the milieu interior which regulates the various metabolic processes at cellular and mitochondrial level for life to be sustained. In gross terms, health is defined as "The state of physical, mental and social well-being and not necessarily the absence of disease and infirmity" (WHO). In fact, at the cellular level, the definition of health should be: "Homeostasis of the cellular ecology and a state where there has not been an inordinate loss, reversible or irreversible, of the structural and or functional reserves of the body." Sickness or disease, therefore, can be defined as: "The structural and/or functional abnormality with the implication that the abnormality produced has the potential of lowering the quality of life contributing to a disabling illness or leading to death." Disturbances in environment, including air pollution, adversely affect health in general and the heart in particular.

Heart Diseases and Environment

A heart disease is not necessarily the gift of genes but largely due to the effects of environmental factors, including: (1) *Air pollution* (2) *Nutritional factors* — both over - and under-nutrition and (3) *Psychological behaviour factors*, like hostility and negative emotions such as anger, greed, undue desires, materialistic attachments and maladjustment to daily challenges of life.

While psycho-social factors and living habits such as over-nutrition, smoking and sedentary lifestyles are more related to coronary heart diseases and hypertension, living in overcrowded environment coupled with poor nutrition is responsible for higher incidence of rheumatic fever and rheumatic heart disease which still has a high prevalence in India, while diseases of affluence like hypertension and coronary heart disease have also invaded us in an epidemic form. Control over environmental factors, including the food we eat, the water we drink and the air we breathe, will go a long way to manage and prevent many of the cardiovascular disorders.

Hippocrates, the father of medicine (6th century B.C.), had wisely stressed the role of environment on health when he had stated, "Whoever wishes to study medicine well, should proceed thus: In the first place to consider *The Seasons* of the year .... *The Waters* .... *The Ground* and the *Mode* in which the inhabitants live and what are their pursuits, whether they are fond of *eating* and *drinking to excess* and given to *sedentary living* or they are fond of *exercise and labour*."

A similar sentiment on the relationship of environment to life was expressed by Guru Nanak (1469-1539), when he said, "*Pawan (Air) guru, pani pita, mata dhart muhat, divis raat doi daii daia, khele sagal jagat"* (Air is like God, water is the father and earth is the mother. It is through the harmonious interaction of all these three vital ingredients that the whole universe is being sustained).

Air Pollution and Heart Disease

Without food an adult can survive for three weeks, without water for three days but without air not more than three minutes. So much is the importance of fresh air to life. That is why in our sacred texts, while water is compared to father and earth to mother, air has been equated with God.

The last fifty years have seen a rapid growth in industry, ever-increasing number of transport vehicles and overcrowding of the urban populations. The exhaust from the chemical factories, thermal power stations, motor vehicles and generator sets at houses and business establishments have thrown a large number of pollutants into the environment, which have proved harmful to the human population through the polluted food eaten and the polluted air breathed in, and contact of the chemicals with the skin and eyes. Animal experiments with the long-term effects of atmospheric pollution have demonstrated that the glycolytic processes are intensified, the bioenergetic processes are inhibited and the synthesis of proteins and RNA (Ribose Nucleic Acid) is increased in the myocardium of experimental animals exposed to air pollution. Mostly the toxins in the polluted air affect the lungs, the skin, eyes and kidneys, and are carcinogenic but the cardiovascular system is also affected indirectly or directly by the following harmful elements in the polluted air.

Toxic Elements and Gases
(1) Carbon monoxide (CO), sulphur dioxide (SO_2), nitric dioxide (NO_2), ozone (O_3), lead (Pb), carbon dioxide (CO_2), mercury (Hg) and cadmium (Cd). (2) Suspended Particulate Matter (SPM) (3) smoke-nicotine, hydrocarbons (4) industrial waste (5) unprocessed sewage (6) smog (7) airborne allergens, fungi, viruses and bacteria.

The heart may be damaged by air pollution indirectly, secondary to lung disease (corpulmonale), through changes in the haemoglobin quality with carboxyhaemoglobin due to carbon monoxide, increased occurrence of hypertension (lead, mercury and cadmium), enhanced atherosclerosis and vasospasm (nicotine in cigarette smoking) or increased myocardial damage, coronary disease and congestive heart failure (smog, CO, suspended particulate matter and SO_2).

Carbon Monoxide (CO) and Cardiovascular System
The combining power of CO with haemoglobin is 210 times more than oxygen (O_2). The source of CO is cigarette smoking, vehicular emissions and passive smoking. When carbon monoxide enters the blood, it immediately displaces the oxygen and mixes with the haemoglobin to result in carboxyhaemoglobin which results in damage to all vital organs, the sufferer turns blue, gets asphyxia and as oxygen does not reach the vital organs like the heart and the brain, these may suffer irreversible damage that proves fatal if the carbon monoxide is not immediately replaced with oxygen. Children and elderly people are more vulnerable to this effect. Smokers carry 10-20 per cent carboxyhaemoglobin, depending upon the number of

cigarettes smoked. Symptoms like headache, dizziness, confusion, lassitude and severe breathlessness precede death. Carbon monoxide pollution of air also increases the occurrence of congestive heart failure in the elderly. Preventive strategies against morbidity and mortality from carbon monoxide poisoning should be targeted against vehicular exhaust by strict legislation and by introducing anti-smoking measures at large.

Cigarette Smoke

Tobacco contains about 1500 toxins, including nicotine as the major one. Among others are carbon monoxide, hydrogen cyanide, methane, formaldehyde and several hydrocarbons. General health hazards of cigarette smoking are well known—chronic bronchitis, lung cancer, cancer of voice-box, stomach, urinary bladder and cervix being some of the well recognised ones. The cardiovascular harmful effects of smoking include increased pulse rate, spasm of coronary arteries, angina, myocardial infarction, peripheral arterial disease (Burger's disease is a painful condition of legs often ending in gangrene and loss of limb). Sudden cardiac death is also more common in smokers. Passive smoking through pollution of atmospheric air by the side stream smoke is responsible for 53,000 deaths in the USA. Smoking also results in increased blood fibrinogen levels, blood viscosity and polycythemia, all these factors aggravate coronary heart disease. In our own study from All India Institute of Medical Sciences, smoking was the major risk factor for myocardial infarction in patients below 40 years of age proven to have coronary artery disease on coronary angiography. As cessation of smoking reverses the harmful effect of smoking, including heart disease, anti-smoking campaigns should be put into practice on a war-footing.

Miscellaneous Air Pollutants

Poor air quality due to various pollutants has the potential for serious adverse health effects including the cardiovascular system through perturbances of the cellular ecology over long periods of exposure. In one study from Michigan, USA, air pollution with suspended particulate matter with aerodiameter of 10 microns (PM10) — Particulate Matter 10 — or less was associated with a high daily admissions for ischaemic heart disease specially among the elderly above 65 years of age. Ozone (O_3), which comes from the vehicle exhaust, is also related to high daily mortality in summer, as during that season the ozone levels in air were found to be high, in a study from London. Ozone has toxic effects on bronchi and myocardium. Nitrogen dioxide (NO_2), another pollutant from vehicular emission, mostly the diesel engines, may result in pulmonary oedema and aggravation of coronary disease. Air pollution from sulphur dioxide (SO_2) occurs through coal and wood burning for fuel, thermal power station exhausts and vehicular emissions, more so the diesel exhaust. Toxic effects of SO_2 include impaired lung function and exercise capacity, higher mortality from neoplasms, cardiovascular disease and lung diseases. Air pollution by lead (Pb) occurs through the leaded petrol. Toxic effects of lead pollution include impaired IQ, development defects in children and possibly hypertension. Cadmium has also been reported to be related to pathogenesis of hypertension, possibly by its effect on proximal renal tubules.

Apart from the toxic effects, as detailed above, some of the air pollutants produce a bad odour, highly disagreeable to the sense of smell, and producing a nauseating feeling, thus, indirectly affecting the cardiovascular system through disturbed heart rate and blood pressure, which in turn could aggravate angina, arrhythmias and congestive heart failure or initiate the onset of an acute heart attack.

Temperature Changes

The ideal temperature for a human being is between 20^0 and 25^0C or 68^0 and 77^0F. Temperature extremes results in high morbidity and mortality from cardiovascular disease due to fluid and electrolyte imbalance at high temperatures, and due to increased peripheral resistance and blood pressure at lower temperatures. In a study from the Netherlands, there was a 57 per cent higher cold-related, unexpected mortality at temperatures below 20^0C (68^0F) and an excess of 26 per cent heat-related in expected mortality at temperatures above 25^0C (77^0F). This higher mortality with extremes of temperatures was attributed to cardiovascular causes.

Noise Pollution

Chronic exposure of children to the high level urban traffic noise has been reported to result in higher blood pressures. As the heart rates did not increase, this effect is reported to be due to the increase in peripheral vascular resistance. Environmental noise pollution could thus be a contributing factor to higher prevalence of hypertension in the city dwellers. Preventive strategies against hypertension, therefore, must make note of this observation and accordingly institute desirable measures, especially during childhood.

Delhi has witnessed huge expansion in population, both of the people and of transport vehicles over the last three decades. From a population of 35 lakhs in 1970, it was 86 lakhs in 1990 and it is projected to be 128 lakhs by the year 2000. The number of diesel-driven vehicles increased from 16,658 in 1971 to 75,707 in 1987. A special mention of diesel-driven vehicles is made here, as these are the main source of sulphur dioxide which is responsible for many cardiopulmonary diseases. Although overcrowding is not as big a problem in Delhi as in Calcutta and Bombay, yet aggressive invasion of the green zone around Delhi by massive construction of houses to accommodate the ever-increasing urban migration to the capital of India and the rapidly growing industrial units have resulted in grave ecological imbalance due to environmental pollution.

Despite introduction of strict planning restrictions, there has been a 57 per cent increase in industrial units from a figure of 26,000 in 1971 to 41,000 in 1981. The paradox of "palaces and pollution" is emerging as a new phenomenon in some of the unauthorised residential complexes and farmhouses. Due to non-availability of regular electric supply, the residents have to install heavy generator sets run on diesel, kerosene or petrol. These generator sets are also installed in most of the business establishments. With electricity cuts being so frequent, the use of generators create pollution not only due to noise but also by their exhaust emission containing carbon monoxide, sulphur dioxide, lead, nitrogen dioxide, ozone and particulate matters. There is thus the paradox of airconditioned comfort inside and polluted breathing air outside these houses and shops, using these generator sets. In Delhi, Indraprastha and Badarpur Thermal power plants are reported to be emitting 25,550 tonnes of sulphur dioxide per annum, the projected figure for the year 2000 being 49,000 tonnes per annum. While emissions from domestic sources have remained static over the years, those from industrial and transport sources have significantly increased. Estimated emission of suspended particulate matter follows a pattern similar to that of sulphur dioxide, both being contributed by vehicles and industry. Dust-storms which are quite common in Delhi around May and June, preceding the rains, also greatly contribute to the air pollution with suspended particulate matter. The monthly mean suspended particle concentration in June was 600 microgram (µg)/metre^3, while the WHO guideline is between 150 and 230 microgram (µg)/metre^3. Road transport adds fuel to fire in aggravating the atmospheric pollution with suspended particulate matter. Buses, trucks and tempos in particular are a major source of diesel smoke, and sufferers are essentially the pedestrians, cyclists and those using the two- and three-wheeler transport vehicles. Lead content of petrol largely used in Delhi as supplied from the Mathura refinery is quite high at 1.8 g/L. Calculating from the number of petrol-driven vehicles in Delhi, the estimated annual lead emission is around 6,000 tonnes. Carbon monoxide emission, again whose main source is vehicular transport, has increased from 14,000 tonnes per annum in 1980 to 265,000 tonnes per annum in 1990 in the city of Delhi, and it is estimated to reach 400,000 tonnes per annum by the year 2000. Oxides of nitrogen follow a similar trend to carbon monoxide, and NO_2 emissions in Delhi were 73,000 tonnes in 1990, thermal power stations and vehicles being the major source. Ozone (O_3) has not been generally monitored in Delhi, but the climate of this city is favourable for ozone formation. Oxides of nitrogen and hydrocarbon emissions are also feared to be increasing dramatically and it is likely that ozone may become a serious air pollutant in Delhi in the next decade if timely preventive measures are not taken.

Prevention and Control of Air Pollution

As the sources of air pollution are industrial, vehicular and domestic (indoor), the preventive strategies therefore have to be focussed at these three levels.

Industrial Air Pollution

This can be controlled by strict legislation recommending the height of chimneys and provision of industrial filters for the exhaust that is produced in the thermal power stations and other industries using coal, diesel, wood, kerosene or other fuels as energy source. Industrial units using such fuel should not be allowed to be run in the residential areas. Knowledge of protective devices against chemical warfare may be extended in planning of preventive strategies against urban air pollution.

Vehicular Pollution

In some countries, the transport media are still cycles, two- or three-wheelers, rickshaws and a large number of people walk to their places of work, like in our country. These city dwellers are prone to get maximum effect of air pollution from vehicular traffic run on diesel and leaded petrol. A periodic check of

Domestic (Indoor) Pollution

the vehicles and punishment for the defaulters is the only solution to control vehicular air pollution.

Passive cigarette smoke, stoves, and use of generator sets run on kerosene, petrol or diesel are the sources of indoor air pollution. Strongly discouraging cigarette smoking, use of electric inverters in place of generators and keeping the generator sets at higher places, and providing adequate air filters should be recommended for control of indoor pollution.

Deforestation of the rural areas surrounding the large cities to provide houses for the ever-increasing urban migrations has disturbed the ecology and health relationship between the fauna and flora and human population. Growing of more trees will restore this healthy relationship, thereby preventing many disorders caused by air pollution.

"Smoking is injurious to health" is well-recognised and advertised all over the world. What we need to propagate now is that in big cities like Calcutta, Bombay and Delhi, even "breathing is becoming injurious to health." If adequate preventive measures against air pollution are not thought of and put into practice *now*, then even breathing in certain highly polluted areas may become "lethal to health".

7
ROLE OF THE SPOUSE IN HEART CARE

To resist the frigidity of old age one must combine the body, the mind, and the heart. And to keep these in parallel vigour one must exercise, study, and love.

— CHARLES VICTOR DE BONSTETTEN

It is not merely long life, but a productive long life, useful to the family and the world around us that makes a meaningful living.

Interspouse relationship has a great bearing not only on the couple's health and longevity, but also on the happiness and well-being of the entire family unit. The ramifications and effects of a good and a bad interspouse relationship often extend much beyond the domestic domain and may influence the output at work—both of individuals and business organisations.

In the Indian context, the *Ardhangani* and *Ardhaneshwar* or the wife-husband team have been compared to the two wheels of a chariot of married life. If one of the two wheels is unbalanced, the other automatically gets damaged, thereby shortening the lifespan of the chariot and adversely affecting the aim of *grhastha ashrama*, i.e., the attainment of : (1) *dharma* (virtue) (2) *artha* (worldly desires) and (3) *sukha* (happiness). It is the balanced working of these two wheels in unison that determines the outcome of the quality of life and its longevity.

Health has been defined by the World Health Organisation (WHO) as *a state of physical, mental and social well being and not merely the absence of disease or infirmity*. For a holistic definition of health, the additional words of *spiritual* well-being and *happiness* are most appropriate, especially in the Indian context, where spirituality has been the strong backbone of our ancient culture. The oriental philosophy stressed not only on long life but a productive and useful life in the service of others.

Saints, *yogis* and *rishis* are but among the very few ones who may be living in *ashrams* and the Himalayas to achieve spiritual fulfilment. For the majority of the people in general, the social, mental and spiritual well-being and happiness have to be achieved while performing their normal duties as family members and discharging the duty of a *grhasthi*. Our sages and saints have preached that a true *karmayogi* is the one who discharges his duties to the best of his/her abilities as a *loving spouse*, as *an affectionate and caring parent*, and as an *effective performer* in his/her profession. Living in the world and aspiring to do your optimum best for the community and for the country, in whatever field you are, is the real *bhakti* and not renouncing the world and seeking shelter in jungles and the Himalayas to achieve *Nirvana*. Swami Vivekananda had said: "Those who live for others really live, those who live only for themselves are more dead than alive."

Before we talk of the specific role of the spouse in heart care and longevity, let us see the connection of the spouse to total health care and long life. As health is not merely the absence of disease or infirmity but a state of physical, mental, social and spiritual well-being, how does then one achieve all the wonderful ingredients of health, single-handed by oneself or with someone's help? One can eat well, dress well, go about in social circles, read literature for better communication with others and go to religious places for spiritual lessons and thus try to achieve most of the components of health. Doing it single-handed, however, appears a herculean task—in the company of the partner, you do it effortlessly. Imagine if the other partner is not exposed to the same degree physically, mentally, socially and spiritually; the balance will not be proper and there will be repeated occasions and a tendency for a complex developing between the spouses. If either one develops a superiority complex and the other starts feeling inferior, the result is the same — a disturbed equilibrium and strains developing in the pious interspouse relationship, thereby, adversely affecting the environment at home as well as the working milieu at the job. This disturbed environment is then responsible for deterioration in the quality of life and possibly in its shortening too. A perfect interspouse relationship, understanding and solving each other's problems is, therefore, mandatory for attaining the perfect state of health of both the members of this *ardhanareshwar-ardhangini* team, as a harmonious interspouse relationship will lead to enhancement in the quality of life and possibly its lengthening also. One member being in perfect shape of physical, mental and social status will not get him/her that much happiness and enjoyment, compared to when both have the same degree of achievement in these three components of health — this is possible by an active, positive attitude in interspouse help and total absence of misunderstanding.

Apart from the role in health care in general, a spouse has a major positive role for heart care in particular at the following three levels. A non-harmonious interspouse relationship on the other hand could play a negative role in the well-being of heart of either or both. The various aspects of the positive role of the spouse in heart care are :
1) Prevention of heart attack.
2) During recovery from a heart attack.
3) During the phase of rehabilitation after heart attack.

Prevention of Heart Attack
Heart attacks are occurring at younger ages, practically one-third of the total heart attack patients in India are in their forties and earily fifties. As majority of these victims are men, so the major responsibility falls on the wife when we talk of the role of the spouse in heart care. Prevention of any disease is best achieved by avoiding or eradication of the causative agent of that disease or taking a vaccination against that disease. Unfortunately, in the case of heart attacks, we neither know the causative agents of this disease, nor is there any vaccination against heart attacks either! What we know are some of the *risk factors*, which if present, make the person more prone to heart attacks. These risk factors are: (1) cigarette smoking (2) high blood pressure (3) high blood cholesterol and other blood lipids (4) low levels of HDL (5) lack of physical exercise (6) diabetes mellitus (7) obesity and (8) repeated episodes of being under mental tension and anger.

Smoking

Most of the well-educated people know about the causative role of this risk factor for heart attacks, so being told in an aggressive, authoritative way by any family member, and specially by the wife, is not really appreciated by the person for whose well-being this is being told. So the message should come in a very gentle, affectionate yet persuasive manner to take note of this serious risk factor and discuss the approach to prevention accordingly. Even passive cigarette smoking is harmful to health in general and the heart in particular, and hence, one should avoid sitting in an environment of smoking.

Blood Pressure

This can be kept under control, and prevention of high blood pressure is possible by: (1) Regular physical exercise. (2) Avoiding excess salt comsumption. (3) Limiting alcohol intake to not more than two ounces of whisky, two glasses of wine or two glasses of beer in a day. (4) Avoiding being overweight, by keeping control on excessive eating and drinking and doing regular physical exercises. (5) Mental relaxation through practice of yoga, meditation, music, and attending religious congregations. (6) When drugs are used to control high blood pressure, their periodic monitoring for side-effects is essential, as some antihypertensive drugs lower sexual performance, while others may adversely affect blood sugar, uric acid, cholesterol, and some may give rise to cough, muscle fatigue, nightmares or bronchospasm.

Cholesterol

Effective cholesterol-lowering drugs in the form of Gemfibrozil and Statins are available, but initially all efforts should be made to lower cholesterol by non-drug measures such as:

(1) Controlled Diet

A diet minus fatty foods and sweets. Dietary cholesterol intake should also be lowered; one egg yolk has 300 mg cholesterol and most organ meats are very rich in cholesterol, like liver, kidney etc.; the richest being the brain. Also avoid milk and dairy products, when dietary efforts are being made to lower the cholesterol. Nuts and dry fruits do not contain cholesterol but their excess consumption gives more calories and thus a tendency for overweight.

(2) Exercises

Regular physical exercises help not only in reducing weight but also lower blood cholesterol and triglycerides — both are strong risk factors for heart attacks. Regular physical exercise increases HDL (High Density Lipoprotein) which is the friendly cholesterol that helps in prevention of heart attacks.

Mental Tension Management

Mental tension keeps the blood pressure and heart rate high and may also result in irregularities of the heart beat. It has a major role in causation and aggravation of heart attacks. In ayurveda, it is stated that all those who wish to protect their heart and its roots (coronary arteries) must always avoid all that causes them mental affliction. It is mandatory that the spouse must avoid creating those situations that cause anger and mental tension. The spouse, therefore, has a major role to look into those situations or events that cause mental tension to his/her life-partner and try to prevent such happenings in order to prevent heart attack in the person who is so dear and important to her/him, i.e., the life-partner. Finding a common interest in indoor games, some hobby and music also will bring a great deal of mental relaxation not only to both but to other family members too.

During a Heart Attack

When a heart attack has occurred, the victim has several fears: (1) Fear of a sudden death. (2) Fear of another attack. (3) Fear of losing his job. (4) Fear of sub-optimum performance — physically and sexually after recovery from the heart attack. (5) Fear of decrease in overall productivity.

Although the main treatment for heart attacks is being done by the attending doctor, the spouse has to play a major role in the recovery from this painful stroke by: (a) not being panicky (b) reassuring the patient that all is being effectively taken care of at home during his stay in the hospital, and the colleagues and employers/employees also have been very understanding and cooperative (c) one should not enter into lengthy discussions with the patient in the hospital, and most of the visitors should not be with the patient for more than a few minutes — except the spouse and children who should spend enough time with the patient during the recovery phase after a heart attack, but avoid any argument, debate or a serious discussion.

During Rehabilitation Phase

Rehabilitation after a heart attack starts within the next three to four days in most of the cases which do not have any of the complications and a large number of patients are back home in about two weeks. Starting with the hospital phase, the spouse must sit with the physician and the dietician to note down the instructions to be followed after the patient goes home. There will be some special instructions to the spouse and the patient for later procedures, like balloon angioplasty or bypass surgery. These should be clearly understood by the spouse so that minor adjustment in medication may be done at home itself, instead of rushing to the hospital every time some clarification in treatment is called for.

Normal sexual function may be resumed in most of the cases four to six weeks after recovery from an uncomplicated case of heart attack and about 6-8 weeks after bypass surgery. Some of the medicines may impair the sexual performance, and some patients become very irritable after heart attacks or bypass surgery. The spouse, therefore, should frankly discuss all such and other related problems with their physicians for optimum performance by those who have suffered a heart attack. Most of the patients after a heart attack do get back to their full productive career.

An understanding and caring spouse can be of great help not only in early recovery from a heart attack of her/his partner, but also goes a long way in the prevention of a heart attack by closely sharing and taking the various steps as outlined in this text. It is through harmonious interspouse relationship only that one can hope to achieve a purposeful long life. Prevention of the most common killer disease of modern times, i.e., the heart attack and subsequent recovery becomes very quick with the help and active cooperation of a caring spouse.

8
DRUGS, DEVICES AND DEVOTION IN HEART CARE

So long as you are learning you are not growing old. It's when a man stops learning that he begins to grow old.

— JOSEPH HERGESHEMER

Drugs, *devices* and *devotion* are the three essential ingredients for medical management of the sick in general, and for heart patients in particular. Why particularly heart patients have to be given more importance stands to reason as "heart attack" is more scaring to the patient and the family and the situation demands quick, practically instant availability of the physician for effective treatment of the victim. This, in fact, is true also as by the early institution of treatment, specially the thrombolytic therapy (clot busters) and primary angioplasty (ballooning), many lives can be saved from among those who suffer an acute heart attack. A sudden death outside the hospital, after a heart attack, occurs frequently due to delay in reaching the hospital. The earliest the intervention, whether by drugs or devices, for patients of acute heart attacks, the better are the results in saving more such victims and in minimising heart damage. *Availability*, *behaviour* and *competence* have always been considered as the ABC of a good physician, and this again applies more to the physicians attending to the cardiac patients.

In the modern era of medicine, competence of a physician is the result of his knowledge and practice of latest in drugs and the various devices used in the diagnostics and therapeutics of patient care. Over and above the grasp of knowledge in drugs and devices, the third element which is required as a catalytic agent to complete this reaction of making a perfect physician is the element of devotion. Devotion, in fact, is an integral part of competence and without devotion, competence cannot fully manifest itself. Lack of devotion at times brings a bad name to the noble medical profession, as its nobility lies in committed service to preserve and promote life itself. Even among the *Vedas*, the *Ayurveda* is considered supreme as this treatise deals with the human health care without which we can neither study nor preach or practise the other *Vedas*.

Drugs and Devices for Heart Care

Various types of efficacious drugs are now available for treatment of heart patients depending upon the nature of a malady. The diseases of heart can basically be grouped as: (1) Those involving the valves resulting in their narrowing or incompetence, that commonly occurs due to rheumatic fever in childhood. (2) Heart ailments due to holes in the walls of heart chambers or obstructions to flow of blood from the right-sided chambers to the lungs and the left-sided chambers to the whole body. These defects are usually present at birth and are called congenital cardiac malformations. These disorders as well as the valvular deformities are more amenable to devices (described below) and surgical treatment (discussed in a separate chapter) than to drug therapy. (3) Heart diseases due to irregular, fast or slow heartbeats (arrhythmias). While effective anti-arrhythmic drugs are available for treatment of tachyarrhythmias (fast rhythms), the slow rhythm disorders (bradyarrhythmias) are best treated by using pacemakers. There are now special devices available that can take care of both the tachy and bradyarrhythmias (implantable cardioverter difibrillators). While antiarrhythmic drug therapy may have to be given for a long time, it is mandatory that these patients should be followed under close observation for any clinical side effects, and adverse ECG changes. Patients on long term drug therapy for arrhythmias should have a periodic Holter study done to ascertain that the drug does not have a proarrhythmic effect, i.e., causing arrhythmias other than that for which the drug is being used.

(4) Ischaemic heart disease (coronary artery disease), such as chronic stable angina or unstable angina, and myocardial infarction (heart attack). This heart disease is the result of narrowing of coronary arteries that supply nourishment and oxygen to the heart muscle, due to a pathological process called atherosclerosis. The exact cause of this process is still not known, but risk factors like smoking, high blood cholesterol, hypertension, diabetes, obesity and lack of physical activity appear to either initiate and/or aggravate atherosclerosis. In this heart disease, the patient suffers from severe chest pain at rest or during work or exertion, due to lack of optimum blood supply to the heart muscle. The drugs that are beneficial in this type of heart disease are those that either (1) increase the coronary blood supply such as nitrates and calcium channel blockers or (2) decrease cardiac work and

relieve congestion in heart, such as betablockers, nitrates, calcium channel blockers and angiotensin converting enzyme (ACE) inhibitors, and (3) drugs that work at blood platelets and myocardial cellular level to decrease platelet aggregation (to inhibit clotting of blood) or to improve heart muscle function by direct action such as trimetazidine.

Drugs
When the heart muscle becomes feeble or sluggish in action due to the various diseases mentioned as above or due to direct toxic effect of viruses, bacteria, alcohol or systemic disorders such as diabetes and hypertension, the heart enlarges and loses its function to supply adequate blood for the body needs. This condition is termed as congestive heart failure as it results in swelling of the body and congestion in the lungs, causing severe breathing difficulty. The drugs used for patients suffering from congestive heart failure include digitalis which is like a tonic for the tired heart, diuretics that relieve congestion by bringing out fluid through excessive urination, and once again the drugs that relieve load from the heart by their peripheral vasodilatory (vascular relaxation) effect such as nitrates and ACE inhibitors. As diuretics cause vitamin B complex and potassium depletion, so patients receiving long term diuretic therapy must be supplemented with B complex vitamins and oral potassium. Anorexia, nausea, vomiting and slow pulse rate are the side effects of digitalis (drug to augment heart function) group of drugs, and diuretics may cause muscle weakness and fatigue, nitrates give rise to headache while altered taste sensation and cough may be the side-effects of ACE inhibitors.

Potent drugs for treatment of high blood pressure include diuretics, betablockers, alphablockers, calcium antagonist and ACE inhibitors. Patients taking antihypertensive drugs for a long time should periodically get their blood lipids and serum electrolytes checked.

Devices

There have been rapid advances in the treatment of heart patients in the last three decades. Twenty years back, if a patient with severe angina did not respond to drug therapy, he was advised to undergo coronary bypass surgery. At present, the scene is quite different. Most patients with angina due to obstructive coronary disease are being helped with devices like balloon angioplasty and stent insertions instead of undergoing open heart surgery. These devices have helped patients to go home after one or two days of hospitalisation instead of a few weeks' stay in hospital if they had to undergo open heart surgery. Other examples of devices which have helped cardiac patients are the balloon valvotomies of narrowed heart valves, specially, the mitral valve which is the commonest valvular disease — for this patients were hospitalised for over a week when they were undergoing heart operations. Presently, such patients are being subjected to balloon valvotomies, whether it is narrowed mitral, pulmonary, aortic or tricuspid valve and the patients are sent home the next day. They can resume their job soon after being discharged from the hospital.

Apart from ballooning of the coronary arteries and narrowed valves, angioplasty is done for other vessels also like those of limbs, abdomen and lung. Some patients of high blood pressure due to narrowed renal arteries or the aorta can get permanent cure from hypertension with the use of ballooning devices. Even impotence in the male in some cases has been successfully treated by balloon angioplasty of the pudendal artery and other arteries that supply blood to the genitalia. Stents placed in the blood vessels after balloon dilation help in maintaining long term patency to ensure adequate blood flow across the treated vessels. In patients with holes in heart there are special devices to close these defects without undergoing heart surgery. Some patients of atrial septal defect, ventricular septal defect and patent ductus arterious, depending upon the size of defect, can be cured now with these devices without surgery. Coils of various shapes and sizes are being used to control blood flow in large collateral blood vessels that are found in some patients with congenital cardiac defects who have abnormal arterio-venous communications. Introduction of various types of devices over the last two decades have revolutionised therapeutic approaches for cardiac patients and have not only added more years to their life, but have also brought significant improvement in their overall quality of living.

Devotion in Heart Care and the Doctor's Dilemma
Mere availability of modern drugs and devices do not suffice for optimum health care or heart care. You need the third invisible ingredient, and that is the devotion of the physician handling these devices and other therapeutic interventions. Simply five-star buildings and equipment therein do not necessarily make a good hospital. It is the dedicated workers inside these

complexes that bring out the maximum and productive results out of these establishments. This third dimension has to be seriously borne in mind now as many new medical and "research" centres are presently coming up in the country, especially in cardiology and cardiac surgery. Devotion in general is an integral part of any job to be done well, but it is particularly so in the care of the sick and more so the heart patients, as the urgency considered here is of a much higher degree. This puts the doctors dealing with this speciality on the horns of a peculiar dilemma—the paradox of their preachings and self-care, including care of their family. The physician advises his patients to do regular physical exercise and mental relaxation courses but finds no time himself to do those! The demands on him by virtue of the nature of disease he has to deal with are so heavy and untimely that often it becomes difficult to comfortably accommodate all those who need his help. This results in earning a few enemies even though sincerely worshipping the goddess of devotion. The person who calls on the physician late at night due to his own urgent need is unaware of the fact that his doctor has just returned home after attending a serious emergency and has not even so far had his dinner. Well, dedication and devotion to duty takes him back to attend the emergency either in the operating room, intensive cardiac care unit or the patient's home, with an apple or a piece of bread in hand as his mobile dinner! How is the present mobile cellular culture going to help or harm this balance between demands and devotion remains yet to be seen, but the wonder drugs, the miracle devices and the state-of-the-art equipment will yield positive results only when supplemented by total dedication and devotion. Devotion, I feel, is the small price for getting the medical profession christened as the noble profession. In medical profession duty has to be supplemented by dedication and devotion in order to fulfil the mission of a true healer to give complete relief to the sick and to preserve and promote health.

9
AYURVEDA AND HEART CARE

The true way to render age vigorous is to prolong the youth of the mind.

— MORTIMER COLLINS,
The Village Comedy, i. 56

The word *Ayurveda* stands for knowledge of life and longevity, (*ayus*—age, life, longevity, and *veda*—*vidya* or knowledge). While allopathy (modern medicine), homoeopathy, etc., are the systems of medicine, ayurveda is beyond one system. It is the science and knowledge of life as a whole and it mostly deals with the preservation and promotion of health and prevention of disease (*rasayana*), rather than only aiming at curing of diseases. In fact, it is stated in ayurveda that "Starting treatment when disease has erupted is like starting preparing arms when the war has already been declared." Whether for general medical care or for cardiac care (*hridyarog*), most of the text in several volumes of *Charaka Samhita* (600 B.C.), which is the modern available treatise on ayurveda, has dealt with the preventive aspects of health care:

"From promotive health care, one attains longevity, memory, intelligence, freedom from disorders, youthful age, excellence of lustre, complexion and voice, optimum strength of physique and sense organs, successful words, respectability and brilliance. Rasayana (promotive treatment) means the way for attaining excellent life."

Cardiology and Ayurveda

William Harvey (1578-1657) is credited with the discovery of circulation of blood which he reported in 1628 in his famous monograph *"De Motu cardis et Sanguinis in Animalibus"*. However, we find in *Charaka Samhita* (600 B.C.) a detailed description of heart, its branches, the importance of heart for the whole body, and various therapeutic and preventive approaches for heart care. The heart in the ayurvedic texts, has been compared to the central girder of a building which supports the entire structure. "The human body consisting of six components (four limbs, trunk and head) the Indriyan, the wisdom, the mind, the mental concept and the soul, all of these are dependent upon the normal functioning of the heart."

— *Charaka Sutra 30/4*

During the era, when ayurveda was at its peak, the human body must have been studied at length as there is a detailed description of heart, its roots (the coronary arteries) and various rhythm disorders in the form of *manduka gati* (frog jumps), *ashwa gati* (horse gait), *ustra gati* (camel gait) and *aja gati* (goat leaps). This comparison of the rate, rhythm and flow of radial pulse with that of the gait of animals suggests early recognition of cardiac arrhythmias in ayurveda, much earlier than Harvey, Galen and Roman physicians who might have borrowed this knowledge from India.

"Tremors, cardiac cramps, pause in cardiac beat, stupor, sensation of void in cardiac region, fast heartbeat and exceedingly severe pain are the symptoms of heart disease due to Vata."

—*Charaka Sutra 17:31*

In ayurveda, the heart has been mentioned as the seat of consciousness, and *Murcha* (syncope) was reported to occur on its injury and death occurred after its severe painful condition. As compared to the above description of syncope in ayurvedic texts (600 B.C.), it is worth noting what Robert Adams wrote about syncope in 1827. "In these cases, apoplexy (syncope) must be considered less a disease in itself than symptomatic of one, the organic seat of which was the heart," a description similar to that seen in ayurvedic texts.

William Heberden (1710-1801), an English physician, defined angina pectoris for the first time in modern medicine, but in ayurveda, angina has been termed as *hrishool* and its description goes like this: "The person suffering from Hrishool (angina pectoris) feels as if a heavy stone is kept in the centre of chest and he experiences profuse sweating and vomiting."

— *Sushruta-Nidan*

Maybe some of those patients had advanced to have acute myocardial infarction as profuse sweating and vomiting are mentioned. The pathogenesis of angina was ascribed to an imbalance between blood and air (oxygen) supplied to the heart.

Although blood pressure was first measured by Reverend Stephan Hales (1677-1761), in the carotid artery of a horse, hypertension and its pathogenesis was described in a unique way by Sushruta as *Sira-Kunchan* and *Rakta-Poornata:* "The wind/air contained in the blood vessels produces pain and constriction of arterioles and venules due to provocation and thus raises tension of blood from within."

— *Sushruta-Nidan 1/27*

While the aetiology of many cardiovascular disorders is still not clear to us and we often talk of risk factors, the following descriptions from *Ayurveda* are noteworthy:

"The body fat and flesh increase by avoiding physical exercise and seasonal purification, by excessive indulgence in sleep, sedentary habits, laziness and worries and also by intake of flesh eatables, liquors, salty and acidic articles."
— *Charaka Sutra 17/78-79*

The usefulness of physical exercise is described as follows:

"By physical exercise one gets firmness and strength, lightness, capacity to work, tolerance of difficulties, diminution of impurities and stimulation of *AGNI* (digestion and metabolism), one should practise it in moderation."

In the above description of physical exercise we are being told not only the benefits of exercise but also warned against doing it in excess. While overeating has been blamed for causing cardiac disease, the ayurvedic texts also mention the effect of environmental and other related factors during eating.

"Even the wholesome food, also taken in proper quantity does not get digested well due to anxiety, grief, fear, anger, uncomfortable bed and vigil."
— *Charaka Samhita 311:9*

Coming to the curative and therapeutic aspects, Ayurvedic texts laid stress on the quadruple of *physician, drug, attendant* (Nurse) and also the *patient*, in alleviation of disease. A physician has been described to possess excellence in theoretical knowledge, extensive practical experience, dexterity and cleanliness. The attendant or nurse should have knowledge of attendance, loyalty and cleanliness. A patient, in order to be an equal contributor in its treatment, should be having memory, obedience, and fearlessness in providing information regarding his illness. Qualities of the drug mentioned in *Ayurveda* include its abundance, effectiveness, various pharmaceutical forms and exact composition.

Ayurveda is not just another system of medicine, but is also the knowledge of total health care based on the strong pillars of positive and promotive health. The mistake often made is to equate ayurveda with ayurvedic medicines! Although, ayurveda lays emphasis on both preventive and curative aspects yet its strength has been the former, i.e., the preventive and promotive aspects.

Charaka's description of ayurveda is very systematic and in many ways, it surpasses the modern system of medicine. The approach in ayurveda is broad-based, holistic and health-oriented, while that of modern medicine is largely disease-oriented. Modern medicine is only now, to some extent, emphasising on the role of mind in disease (psychosomatic), while ayurveda from times immemorial had envisaged the body (*sharira*) and soul (*atman*) as one whole unit. For attaining total health, all these have to be in unison and in equilibrium, while their disequilibrium results in disease and disability.

Ayurveda in Preventive Cardiology

Coronary artery disease is the major cause of death and disability in adults and elderly, not only in the developed countries but also in the developing world, including India. Curative treatment, which in fact, is the palliative treatment, such as the balloon angioplasty, atheroctomy, stents and bypass surgery, is a very costly affair which neither most of the families nor the states in developing countries can afford. The answer to contain this epidemic of coronary heart disease (heart attack, angina, cardiac failure and sudden cardiac death) thus lies in its prevention. Modern medicine has been stressing the role of lifestyles, including diet, physical exercise and mental relaxation in the prevention of coronary artery disease through reversal, regression and retardation of the atherosclerosis. When the American cardiologist, Dean Ornish, published his studies in the early 1990's on the reversal and regression of atherosclerosis in patients with coronary artery disease, it was acknowledged the world over as a great step in prevention of heart attacks. It is of interest to note that Dr. Ornish, in fact, started his work on the reversal of atherosclerosis through lifestyle changes after he had his lessons from an Indian *yogi*. The concept of these studies on prevention of coronary heart disease through reversal, retardation and regression of atherosclerosis is based on: (1) vegetarian diet (*saatvik aahaar*) (2) regular physical exercise, *yogasanas* and other aerobic exercises and (3) mental relaxation through meditation. These three pillars are the legs of the tripod on which stands the whole philosophy and science of preventive cardiology for the control and prevention of coronary heart disease. The role of diet (*aahaar*), physical exercise (*yogasanas*), mental relaxation and avoiding of mental affliction has been extensively quoted in ayurvedic texts as the modes for prevention of heart diseases.

In the prevention of heart attacks and the role of mind in this aspect, ayurveda has the following message for us: "Those who desire to protect from the adverse effects on their heart, coronary blood vessels and the contents therein, must particularly avoid all that causes affliction of their mind."

— *Charaka Sutra 3:4*

10

YOGA AND THE HEART

If I were running in the stadium, ought I to slacken my pace when approaching the goal? Ought I not rather to put on speed?
— DIOGENES, LAERTIUS, *Diogenes. Sec. 34.*

Yoga stands for the union—coming together of the self (*Atman*), with the supreme (*Parmatman*), and the means or the science that helps in achieving this celestial union, is called *Yoga Shastra*. The origin of yoga, perhaps, cannot be separated from the origin of human race, as all recorded texts in all faiths and religions mention this human desire of mingling of the self with the Supreme through different avenues, the destination being the same. Patanjali (300 B.C.), however, has been credited with systematically recording facts about yoga and putting it through eight successive stages starting with *yama, niyama, asana, pranayama* and *praatyhara* of the *Hatha Yoga* (more related to physical aspects of yoga), leading onto and over-lapping with the three stages of *Rajayoga*, viz., *dharna* (concentration), *dhyana* (meditation) and finally *samadhi* (illumination) related to the state of mind. The initial stages of (*Hatha*) yoga, in fact, are the steps to reach the higher form of (*Raja*) yoga, which ultimately leads to the consequent attainment of liberation through the yogic way of living. Yoga also means restraining of extrovert activities of the mind as a result of which the "self" alludes in its "own form", leading to self-realisation and awakening of latent powers of mind. Once the mind is overpowered and tamed through yoga, it helps to manifest the full potential of the body, thereby developing the personality of the individual in a multi-directional and productive way. At this point of development through yogic practice, there is no hatred, malice or enmity but equilibrium of mind with love, devotion and understanding of the cosmos. Paramahansa Niranjananandji says: "In love there is only one-track mind, there is no other idea in mind." Such is the attainment with yoga.

What has all this to do with the heart? A lot indeed, as we will analyse shortly. The heart is not only a muscular pump with its walls and valves, blood-vessels, and nerves, but it has to be much more than that to continue to beat nonstop for several decades, quite often much beyond the biological age of three scores plus ten years, and in some instances, it is not out even after scoring a century!

The cardiologists consider the heart as the master-organ of the body. Is it really the master or the slave? If the heart is the master then why does it suddenly start shivering merely at the sight of an unfamiliar or undesirable face or the sound of a few unfavourable harsh words? It races up when faced with an untimely telephone call or an odd time doorbell. Its nuts and bolts start rattling and its body may even crack during heated arguments in a meeting or at the misbehaviour of a loved one. These are some of the situations created by an imbalance of the mind, so heart "the great", in fact is slave to the mind. If that is so, then yoga has a lot to do with the functioning of the heart, its well-being, and its protection from diseases.

The major killers of humanity in the present age are the diseases of the heart and those related to high blood pressure. The exact cause of neither heart attacks nor high blood pressure in the adults amongst whom these two diseases take the maximum toll of life, is not known. Though risk factors like obesity, smoking, high cholesterol and hypertension have been correlated with higher incidence of heart attacks, yet that is not the whole truth and there are as many patients of heart attacks which do not have any of these risk factors as those who have one or more of them. *Charka Samhita* (600 B.C.), the best available text on ayurveda has stated: "Those who wish to protect this vital organ, the heart, and its roots (coronary arteries) must avoid scrupulously all that causes mental affliction." In this enunciation from traditional wisdom, thus comes the message of the powerful role of mind in the well-being of human heart and its protection from disease by avoiding mental stress. The best way to train and tame the mind to keep up its equilibrium when facing the stressful situation, is through the practice of yoga and meditation. We also know that those who regularly practise meditation tend to have slower heart rates and lower blood pressure than non-doers. It is the heart rate systolic pressure product (double product) that determines the myocardial oxygen requirement which is directly proportional to the rate pressure product. The higher the double product, the less economical it is for the heart. Persons with higher heart rates have higher incidence of heart attacks, and the less expensive way to keep the blood pressure and the heart rate slow is through yogic practice and meditation instead of medication. Certain drugs like betablockers do the same thing as achieved through the practice of yoga, but at a cost, not only in money but also the side-effects of drugs.

Coronary arterial tone (temporary narrowing of blood vessels) is also regulated by mental stimuli. It is high during stressful situations and doing mental arithmetic and also noted in animals exposed to mental stress. High coronary tone may result in myocardial ischaemia or infarction and angina-like diseases. The practice of yoga, logically should help in decreasing coronary tone as it normalises the balance between sympathetic and parasympathetic systems.

Another observation of recent research has shown that the individuals who have less R-R variability in their continuous ECG recording, have a higher rate of heart attacks and arrhythmias. Normally, there is a slight but imperceptible variability in R-R interval due to a balanced functioning of sympathetic and parasympathetic limbs of autonomic nervous systems. When there is an excessive working of sympathetic system, the R-R variability disappears, the heart rate and blood pressure also rise and these factors prove harmful for the heart.

Most of the studies reported on the effect of meditation and yoga on cardiovascular system have shown a desirable fall in blood pressure and heart rate and it is quite likely that practice of yoga may restore the R-R variability, thus preventing many heart attacks, angina and arrhythmias.

Yoga, thus, is closely related to the well-being of the human heart and with its regular practice, the incidence of heart attacks and high blood pressure can be brought down not only through the control of the mind, but by the improvement in other risk factors too, such as hypertension, sedentary way of living, diet control and cessation of smoking, which automatically occur in persons who practise yoga regularly. The yogic way of living is a superior way of living and enjoying life in the true sense. Yoga is as helpful in heart care as in total health care.

Meditation vs Medication
Meditation focuses on man, as a whole and not only on disease. Meditation considers the very personality of man as the disease. Medicine considers that diseases come to man and then they go—that they are something alien to man. But slowly this difference has diminished and medical science too has started saying, "Do not treat the disease, treat the patient."

This is a very important statement, because this means that disease is nothing but the way of life which the patient lives. Every man does not fall sick in the same fashion. Diseases also have their own individuality, their personality. So deep down, the patient is the root, not the disease.

Medicine catches the diseases in man very superficially; meditation gets hold of man from deep within. In other words, it can be said that medicine tries to bring about the health of a person from the outside; while meditation tries to keep the inner being of a person healthy. Neither can the science of meditation be complete without medicine, nor can the science of medicine be complete without meditation, since man is both body and soul.

In January 1990, US cardiologist, Dean Ornish, presented his findings to the press, later published in the UK medical journal, *The Lancet*. The essence of his findings was spectacular enough for *Time* magazine to report: "By normal standards, the impossible had happened."

What he had done was to take a group of patients with badly furred-up coronary arteries and offer them a programme of meditation, a low-fat vegetarian diet, and moderate exercises. He showed that those who participated in this new programme responded dramatically with extraordinary reductions in symptoms and with demonstrable unfurring of the arteries to their hearts.

What really distinguished this research on meditation from so much of what had preceded it, was the use of hi-tech imaging where the increase in the diameter of these blood vessels could be visualised and measured.

It was not just preventing patients with heart disease from dying, but of reversing the whole process! The bottom line was this: rather than having to undergo dangerous and invasive cardiac surgery, it was now possible to get better results by taking country walks for 30 minutes three times a week, by meditating, and by eating the prescribed low-fat diet. In addition to the low cost sitting quietly and eating your greens could sure beat a Rs. 100,000 bill for bypass surgery or stenting.

In fact, six major cardiology centres in the US are now offering this programme. One such centre is the New York teaching hospital, Beth Israel. An indication of the extraordinary revolution that is in the making can be gleaned from a November 1993 *Business Week* article, where Dr. Steven Horowitz, chief of cardiology at Beth Israel, is quoted as saying of Dean Ornish's programme: "It's almost medical malpractice not to offer it." Parodoxically in India, the birthplace of this approach, the awareness is only now coming up slowly.

When top doctors in the world's most advanced hospitals start saying that it is almost medical malpractice not to offer meditation for heart disease—and more importantly actually prescribed it—the revolution is unstoppable.

Western medical science is rediscovering what the Eastern healing traditions have long known that "health is the harmonious flow of energy within the body and meditation is the way to realise this."

So the critical question is: If meditation supports the harmonious flow of energy within an individual body, would it also support harmony within a body of people? The potential for saving energy now wasted as a result of intra- and inter-personal conflict is obvious. At a time when increasing efficiency and reducing the cost of productivity are regarded as the keys to economic survival, the possible benefits of meditation have not been lost on business community.

The economic implications of not wasting energy through friction, but making it available for creativity, are also beginning to attract the attention of the business media. The leading US business magazine, *Fortune*, in their December 13, 1993 issue, recommended their readers to "pay attention to their inner self", to "meditate", and to get "centred", in order to be "the best". A 1990 poll of nearly 600 "top leaders" in economics, politics and management, was published in Germany's *Capital* magazine where a surprising 60 per cent anticipated that "meditation will play a far bigger role in the future."

Not only is this group realising that meditation may play a role in the health and well-being of their employees, but they are increasingly appreciating that when people work more harmoniously together, the company benefits as much as the people working there.

In its August 22nd, 1994 issue, the *Fortune* magazine even ran a six-page article entitled, "Leaders Learn to Heed the Voice Within". It describes how top business leaders are discovering the benefits of "tolerance for paradox", "intuition", and even "egolessness"—through meditation. In short, what is dawning on the business community is that whether the issue is blocked coronary artery flow or blocked cash flow, meditation is the missing ingredient.

11

OLD AGE, MODERN MEDICINE AND LONGEVITY

Light heart, light foot, light food and slumber light, these lights shall light us to old age's gate.

— EDWARD HOVELL THURLOW

Rapid scientific developments in the medical sciences, specially over the last fifty years, have to a large extent contributed to improving the quality of life and also lengthening the lifespan. Excellent diagnostic aids like CT (Computerised Tomography) Ultra Sonography, Magnetic Resonance Imaging (MRI), Positron Emission Tomography (PET), Electron Microscopy and advances in cytohisto pathologic techniques now help in early and exact diagnosis of several diseases, thereby, helping the sick to get timely and effective treatment. Therapeutic interventions like potent antibiotics and anti-cancer drugs, specific powerful tools and vaccines against communicable diseases such as smallpox, polio, typhoid, cholera and tuberculosis have helped in control of many communicable diseases. Oral rehydration therapy and improved nutritional standards are saving millions of children from malnutrition.

Regular antenatal check-ups and good peripartum (related to the period of pregnancy) and post-natal care and the speciality of neo-natology have significantly decreased maternal and infant mortality.

Intervention procedures like balloon angioplasty, laser, stents, coils, other similar devices and pacemakers for heart patients have given a new lease of life and also enhanced the quality of life for those suffering from heart problems. Wonders of heart and lung transplant, kidney and liver and other organ transplants have made many more people live useful productive lives for longer times than was ever thought possible in the past.

Age has more to do with our attitudes and thoughts than the biological aging alone. As G. Edward put it: *It is not by the gray of the hair that one knows the age of the heart.*

The setting sun of retirement brings with it several psycho-social, personal and health-related problems. To those who feel that the in-service period of power and fame is like a brightly-lit day and the retirement phase of life is like a dark night, I wish to remind them that the beautiful stars that we all enjoy seeing are visible only during the night. Old age is, therefore, another side of the coin with its own beauty and charm. As Cicere, De Senectuta stated : *It is in old men that reason and judgement are found, and had it not been for old men no state would have existed.*

Most countries of the world, being governed by the head of their state beyond 60 years of age, is a testimony to this statement. Depending upon the average life expectancy, the retirement age is variable between 55 years and 75 years in the various countries and also it is job-related, being the lowest in military services and highest for the judiciary. Possibly, aging enhances the fine tuning for right decision making which is so much needed by the judges. *We grow with years more fragile in body but morally stouter, and we can throw off the chill of a bad conscience almost at once,* stated Logan Smith in his book, *After Thoughts*.

Not only in state service but even in family business and corporate services, retirement is essential in order to induct the new talent. Even before the old leaves fall off, they are left behind by the newly growing leaves, this is the law of nature. For the production in an industrial unit to be maintained at the maximum, the old machinery has to be phased out by the new sophisticated one. These are but a few examples with which we are all quite familiar. The coming of monsoon may be unpredictable but the coming of retirement is most certain. If this *rain* of retirement is so certain after the *reign* of authority and power, then why not get fully prepared from all angles such as financial, psycho-social and those related to health, to boldly face and withstand the rainy season of retirement well in advance? Preventive strategies for this phase of life must be planned well in time when sound in position, physique and psyche.

If retirement is inevitable, and sure it is, then why should one be afraid of it? Lucky are those who attain retirement and for that we should be grateful to God. *To know how to grow old is the master work of wisdom and one of the most difficult chapters in the great area of living* (Amiel, *The Journal*, 21 September, 1874). There is great honour and lasting grace in retirement. Staying in chair on extensions by asking is to gather some copper in exchange of gold!

Retirement and Health
The fact of reaching the age of retirement has obviously been due to a reasonably good health.

Having survived beyond the fifth or sixth decade, the diseases that one is likely to encounter are those of the cardiovascular system and cancer. The other diseases in the post-retirement old age may be the degenerative disorders involving the central nervous system, osteoarthritis of joints, cataract, dental problems, and disorders of prostate in the males and of uterus and ovaries in the females. Heart diseases and strokes are the commonest killers as well as responsible for disability in the aged.

Heart Disease and its Management in the Senior Citizens

"We are as old as our arteries", is an old saying. Heart attacks and brain attacks (stroke) being responsible for maximum deaths and disability in the elderly, the modern version of the above quotation could perhaps be rephrased to read, *We are as old as our coronary and cerebral arteries.*

With control over many infectious diseases and eradication of others, such as smallpox with decreased frequency of famines and with improved standards in nutrition, there has been a global increase in the population beyond sixty years of age and several millions now live beyond the biblical age of three scores plus ten.

Magnitude of the Heart Problems among the Elderly

The grey zone of 60-65 years may be considered the zone of post-retirement beyond which people are placed in the category of elderly. According to WHO, by the year 2000, there will be 100 million people over the age of 65 in the developing countries. In India, as per the 1991 census, we had 35 million people above the age of 65 years and by the year 2000, the figure is estimated to be about 50 million. If 60 years is taken as the cut-off line for the elderly, these figures then will be 54 million and 75 million, respectively. These senior citizens face health problems of a different nature. They have obviously withstood successfully the tests of infections, to now enter the arena where they will face the degenerative disorders. Although old age is no immunity to infectious diseases, yet the major causes of mortality and morbidity in the elderly are cancer and cardiovascular diseases.

Cardiovascular Diseases in the Elderly

This is the main cause of death accounting for geriatric mortality. It accounts for nearly over one-third of deaths in the elderly, mainly from coronary disease stroke, and congestive heart failure, the basic process being that of atherosclerosis or hardening of the arteries that supply pure oxygenated blood to the heart, the brain, the kidneys, the viscera and the limbs.

Although we do see some patients with congenital heart diseases such as aortic stenosis and atrial septal defect, and occasional cases of rheumatic valvular lesions in those age above 60, yet the commonest cardiovascular problems seen in the elderly are due to (1) coronary heart disease (heart attacks and angina) (2) hypertension (3) stroke (4) arrhythmias requiring pacemakers or drug treatment (5) congestive heart failure (6) varicose veins and (7) painful claudication of legs due to atherosclerotic narrowing of arteries, thereby hampering blood supply specially when more blood is required, such as during walking (8) weakening of the walls of large arteries and aorta also results in sac-like widening of these blood vessels, the disorder called aneurysms and rupture of one of these may result in loss of consciousness, paralytic stroke and even sudden death. Another type of heart disease seen in association with chronic lung disease in the elderly is the condition of chronic corpulmonale, a condition of right heart failure (leg oedema, liver congestion, cyanosis and congested prominent neck veins), as a result of chronic bronchitis, smoking, or after prolonged exposure to domestic or industrial smoke and fumes.

Special Features for Cardiac Care in the Elderly

1. The elderly often tend to suppress their symptoms, so they should be given a very patient hearing and due importance given to even minor complaints like, "not feeling too bright today", and "profuse undue sweating" could be a manifestation of silent heart attack as painless heart attacks are more common in the elderly, specially among the diabetics.

2. Environmental factors such as sudden changes in temperature, extreme cold or heat have a strong deleterious effect on the cardiovascular function in the elderly, so the senior citizens have to be protected against such exposures in order to prevent frequent occurrence of aggravation of angina, heart attack, tachyarrhythmias (rapid and at times irregular beating of heart) and congestive heart failure.

3. Disease, disability or death of the spouse or a close friend often result in serious disturbances and imbalance in the psychological behaviour of the elderly and this in turn aggravates or initiates serious cardiac malfunction in the elderly. Death within a few months of the demise of the spouse is not uncommon in the elderly.

Special Treatment Considerations for the Elderly

While most of the drugs, devices and surgical procedures used for cardiac patients in general can also be used and are being used successfully in the elderly too, certain therapeutic precautions are worth considering:

(1) Drug clearance is delayed by the kidney and liver in the elderly, so dosages of various drugs should be modified accordingly in amount and frequency of administration.

(2) The elderly as such are hypokinetic in their responses and reactions, so sedatives and tranquillisers should be given in a smaller dosage and under careful monitoring.

(3) Preferably give the least number of drugs with a smaller dosage for short periods.

(4) Except in emergency situations like myocardial infarction complicated with shock or serious arrhythmias where ICCU (Intensive Cardiac Care Unit) treatment and monitoring may be mandatory, the elderly should be preferably treated at home; and while in hospital, a close relation should be permitted to stay with the aged patients.

(5) Surgery: While the elderly are not denied any cardiac operations, they should be carefully evaluated for other organ systems like lung function, kidney status, cerebrovascular status and condition of their prostrate. A satisfactory functioning of all these systems is very necessary for a successful outcome from any heart operations.

(6) Non-cardiac Surgery: The elderly often need surgery for prostrate, cataract, gall-bladder, uterus, dental extractions, etc. It is important that before they go for any major surgery, their blood pressure should

be ascertained in normal range, any arrhythmia, if present, should be treated adequately, and unless it is a dire emergency, routine operations should be postponed until six months after acute myocardial infarction. For a patient with an advanced degree of heart block, a temporary pacemaker lead may be necessary before the patient goes for a major surgery under general anaesthesia. Rarely, if a patient is having severe angina and coronary angiography shows significant disease of one or more coronary arteries, this patient should be first subjected to myocardial revascularisation by either ballooning angioplasty or bypass surgery before any major non-cardiac surgery is undertaken.

(7) Use of Drugs in the Elderly: When using drugs in the elderly for the treatment of hypertension, heart failure or arrhythmias, more close monitoring is needed to see for the various side-effects which may impair their quality of life-like constipation, postural giddiness (due to postural hypotension—low blood pressure), muscle weakness (hyponatremia and hypokalemia), depression (sedatives) and increased frequency of urination (diuretics), thus disturbing their sleep. At the earliest possible, drugs should be reduced and stopped if clinical situation safely permits.

(8) Non-surgical intervention like ballooning angioplasty of coronary and peripheral arteries, and stent implantation may be done in the elderly as successfully as in other patients.

(9) Pacemakers: A large number of the elderly have extended their lifespan by decades with the help of pacemakers. These can be given at any age, making sure that renal and cerebral status of the patient is

satisfactory and there is no evidence of malignancy. Implantable Cardioverter Defibrillators (ICD) are now available, which automatically detect both the fast and slow arrhythmias, and accordingly choose to either give an electric shock to terminate the otherwise fatal arrhythmia (ventricular fibrillation) or work as a pacemaker to restart the normal heart rhythm in cases of complete heart blocks. These devices have proved very useful in survivors of sudden cardiac death victims, i.e., those who have been resuscitated after cardiac arrests.

(10) Rehabilitation: Cure from the cardiac disease may not be possible in all the elderly cardiac patients, so the aim should be to make the best use of their limited cardiac capacity to enable them to enjoy the optimum quality of life in their remaining years. Unfortunately, "interventions" and "modifications" in their dietary and living habits in advanced ages beyond the seventies and the eighties may not be readily welcome by the elderly, and such advice should be given with due care. Mild to moderate regulated physical exercises should be encouraged at any age, but strenuous exercises should be avoided.

Sex in Elderly Heart Patients

Although India has been known for centuries for its widely read sex manual—the *Kamasutra* — and its explicit erotic carvings in the famous temples, yet when it comes for discussion at personal and social levels, then sex becomes taboo. It is said that age does not depend upon years but upon temperament and state of health. Some men are born old and some never grow old. It is also quoted somewhere *that man is as old as he feels and woman as old as she looks*. In the modern age, the looks are certainly being kept in good shape even into the old age, thanks to good nutrition, gyms, beauty parlours, hair dyes and cosmetics! And as far as men are concerned, no one ever likes to feel old. Satisfaction of sexual desire, therefore, is like fulfilling other basic urges such as hunger and sleep. A perfect mutual interspouse understanding will go a long way to accomplish the desired sexual needs. For the elderly afflicted with heart disease certain precautions have to be observed: (1) After a heart attack, a patient could resume sex only when there is no angina or breathlessness on daily routine activities. (2) Those with chronic stable angina should use a nitrate tablet sublingually before the act. (3) Avoid sex for about an hour after a meal. (4) After a bypass surgery, sex may be resumed as soon as the aches and pains are over and there is no angina on usual exertion.

Prevention of Cardiovascular Disease in the Elderly

All preventive measures such as: (1) regular physical exercise (2) control of hypertension by non-drug means and use of drugs (3) avoiding smoking (4) control of blood lipids by dietary measures and (5) mental relaxation with meditation, yoga, religious congregations *(satsang)* and music, that are advocated in general, are applicable to the elderly as well. Even when started in later years, these measures have been shown to regress atherosclerosis and prevent or postpone the occurrence of cardiac events. *Strenuous physical exercises must be avoided in the elderly.* As Charles Victor put it: *To resist frigidity in old age, one must combine the body, the mind and the heart, and to keep these in parallel vigour, one must exercise, study and love.*

In an attempt to cure hypertension or heart disease in the elderly, the physician should not injudiciously use various drugs and devices without looking into the overall outcome of these methods of treatment. Any therapeutic measure used in the elderly must not result in deterioration in his/her quality of life at the cost of a few added years. While *'cure'* from heart disease in the elderly may not be possible, *'care'* of the elderly with a heart disease is certainly possible.

Retirement is not the end of the drama of life but only another episode, starting with a new set-up and some changes in the orchestra and the stage. Several historic contributions in the field of arts, education and culture have come from people who were beyond the so-called age of retirement. So it is never too late as is evident from the following lines of Justice Olivere Wendell Holmes: *To be seventy years young is far more cheerful and hopeful than to be forty years old.*

With longevity comes old age and growing years have their own inherent problems. With enthusiastic preventive measures and excellent curative methods many of us would be attaining old age. For those who think that youth was like a bright day and old age is like a dark night, I have the following few lines to offer:

It is too late! Ah nothing is too late,
till the tired heart shall cease to palpitate.
Cato learned Greek at eighty; Sophocles,
wrote his grand Oedipus, and Simonides,
bore off the prize of verse from his compeers,
when each had numbered more than four score years.
Chaucer at Woodstock with the nightingales,
at sixty wrote the Canterbury Tales;

> Goethe at Weimar, toiling to the last,
> completed Faust when eighty years were past.
> These are indeed exceptions; but they show
> how far the gulf-stream of our youth may flow.
> Into the Arctic regions of our lives ....
> for age is opportunity no less
> than youth itself, though in another dress,
> and as the evening twilight fades away
> the sky is filled with stars, invisible by day.
>
> — Longfellow, *Morituri Salutamus* 1.238

EPILOGUE

Such books have no end. Nor should they have. Search is always a continuing process. Dr. H.S. Wasir's effort to draw man's attention to spiritualism, while discussing cardiac problems, is ceaseless. All of his books do not talk of heart disease but of lack of a holistic approach to life.

As in life, Dr. Wasir emits through his latest book, *Heart Care*, an approach of tolerance, of feeling that all have some share of truth. The reference to all aspects that guard heart against challenges and attacks is incidental. What he tries to convey is that man's faith in cleanliness and godliness is his best armour. All the graces of life are possible only when we learn the art of living nobly.

And as Mahatma Gandhi said: "If love was not the law of life, life would not have persisted in the midst of death." Dr. Wasir's book is a message of defiance, to those who want to fight for longevity.

He is a curious mixture of yogi and doctor. His medicine includes music, meditation and mysticism. He has denied himself even the company of his family but he has produced for heart patients a series of treatise on how to live in a style in the midst of stress and strain.

Kuldip Nayar
Journalist, Writer and Former High Commissioner of India to U.K.

GLOSSARY OF MEDICAL TERMS

ACE : Angiotensin Converting Enzyme — An enzyme required for genesis of angiotensin — a powerful blood vessel constrictor.
Aneurysm: circumscribed dilation of an artery
Angina: cardiac chest pain
Angiography: radiography of vessels after the injection of a radioplaque solution
Angioplasty: reconstruction of a blood vessel by ballooning
Angiotensin: a potent vasoconstrictor
Anorexia: diminished appetite, aversion to food
Aortic Stenosis: narrow aortic valve
Arrhythmia: irregular rhythm of heart
Arteriole: a terminal artery
Asphyxia: impaired or absent exchange of oxygen and carbon dioxide
Atherectomy: removal of fatty deposit in blood vessel
Atherogenesis: narrowing of arteries
Atherosclerosis: particularly blocked arteries due to fat deposition
Atherosclerotic Plaques: fatty streaks
Atrial Septal Defect: hole in the partition between the upper two chambers — atria — of heart
Bronchospasm: constriction of air passages
CABG: Coronary Artery Bypass Graft
Carboxyhaemoglobin: stable union of carbon monoxide with haemoglobin

Carcinogenic: cancer-producing substance
Cardiomyopathy: flabby heart muscle or heart muscle disease
Cardiovascular: relating to the heart and blood vessels
Cerebrovascular: relating to blood vessels of the brain
Chemotherapy: treatment of disease by drugs
Cholesterol: one of the blood fats — dissolved in blood
Claudication Pain: diminished blood supply to the limbs causing pain in legs on walking
Coronary Arterial Tone: temporary narrowing of blood vessels
Corpulmonale: heart disease secondary to lung disease
CT: Computerised Tomography
Cyanosis: deficient oxygenation of the blood leading to a dark bluish or purplish coloration of the skin
Digitalis: Drug to augment heart function
Diuretics: drugs that result in frequent urination
Endophrine: substance akin to morphine
Homeostasis: the state of equilibrium in the body with respect to various functions and chemical compositions of the fluids and tissues
Hyperinsulnemia: excessive insulin in blood
Hypertension: high blood pressure
Hypokalemia: an abnormally low concen-tration of potassium in the circulating blood
Hyponatremia: abnormally low concentration of sodium ions in the circulating blood
Hypotension: low blood pressure
ICCU: Intensive Cardiac Care Unit
Leg Oedema: swelling of feet and legs
Liver Cirrhosis: disease of the liver leading to body swelling and internal bleeding
Lp (a): lipoprotein (a)

Glossary

MRI: Magnetic Resonance Imaging

Myocardial Infarction: heart attack

Myocardial Revascularisation: re-establishment of blood supply to the heart.

Myocardium: the middle layer of the heart, consisting of the cardiac muscle

Neurohumoral Activity: activity related to the nervous system and the endocrine system

Osteoarthritis: degenerative joint disease

Patent Ductus Arterious : abnormal communication between the aorta (main blood vessel carrying pure blood for the whole body) and the pulmonary artery (main blood vessel carrying impure blood to the lungs).

Peripartum: related to the period of pregnancy

Prophylaxis: prevention of disease

Psychosomatic: of mind and body as a unit

Pulmonary Oedema: waterlogging in the lungs

Radiotherapy: use of electromagnetic or particulate radiations in the treatment of disease

Renal : related to kidneys

Splanchnic: related to abdominal organs

Stents: small wire coils used to maintain normal blood flow in the ballooned blood vessels.

Syncope: transitory loss of consciousness or blackouts

Tachyarrhythmias: rapid and at times irregular beating of heart.

Triglycerides: another blood fat like cholesterol

Ultrasonography: location, measurement or delineation of deep structures by ultrasonic waves.

VLDL Very Low Density Lipoprotein — They carry blood triglycerides.

Valvoplasty: opening of narrow stenotic valves

Vasospasm: temporary narrowing of blood vessels
Ventricular Septal Defect: hole in the partition between lower (muscular) chambers (ventricles) of heart

INDEX

abdomen, 80
accidents, 23, 41, 42
acids, 35; mono-unsaturated fatty, 33; poly-unsaturated fatty, 33
Adams, Robert, 86
addiction, 41, 49
After Thoughts, 100
aging (old age), 14, 52, 98-109
AIDS, 21, 22, 23, 42
air pollution, 58; airborne allergens, 60; and heart disease, 59-63; carbon monoxide, 60-61; cigarette smoke, 61; industrial, 66; pollutants, 62-63; prevention and control of, 66-67; toxic elements and gases, 60; vehicular, 66
alcohol, 8, 11, 23, 24, 28, 31, 35, 41-42, 49, 56, 70, 79
Alcott, Amios Bronson, 30
All India Institute of Medical Science (AIIMS), 45, 49, 61
allopathy, 84
alphablockers, 80
Amiel, 100
anemia, 3, 4, 5, 7
angina, 4, 6, 8, 19, 23, 43, 45, 51, 61, 63, 78, 80, 86, 89, 93, 102, 103, 105, 107; pain, 3
angiography, 55, 105
angioplasty, ballooning, 4, 20, 25, 36, 55, 75, 76, 80, 81, 88, 99, 105
Angiotensin Converting Enzyme (ACE) inhibitors, 4, 6, 79, 80

angiotensin, 4, 79
anorexia, 79
antiarrhythmic drugs, 78
antihypertensive treatment, 36, 54, 56, 72, 80
aorta, 55, 80, 102
aortic stenosis, 102
aortic valve, 5, 6, 7, 80
apoplexy, 86
arrhythmia, 3, 5, 6, 19, 41, 45, 63, 78, 85, 93, 102, 104, 105, 106
arteries, 46, 81, 95, 100, 102; blocked, 27, 97; carotid, 86; hardening of, 44, 102; prudendal, 81
arterioles, 35; constriction of, 86
artherogenesis, 46, 47
asana, 8, 15, 17; *Ganeshasana*, 17; *Padmasana*, 15, 16; *Pranayam*, 16; *Shavasana*, 15, 16, 17; *Siddhasana*, 15, 16; *Yoganidra*, 17
asphyxia, 60
aspirin, 4
atherectomy, 4, 36, 88
atherosclerosis, 4, 9, 23, 27, 31, 32, 44, 46, 60, 78, 89, 102, 107
atherosclerotic plaques, 31
atrial septal defect, 81, 102
ayurveda, 20, 21, 25, 29, 48, 73, 77, 89, 92; and cardiology, 85-88; and heart care, 84-89; in preventive cardiology, 88-89;

bacteria, 60, 79
betablockers, 4, 36, 47, 79, 80, 92

Beth Israel, 95
blood fibrinogen levels, 61
blood lipids, 31, 32, 45, 71, 80, 107; High Density Lipoprotein (HDL), 31, 50; lipoprotein (Lp), 31; Low Density Lipoprotein (LDL), 31, 48; Triglycerides, 31, 46, 48; Very Low Density Lipoprotein (VLDL), 31, 48
blood platelets, 45, 79
blood polycythemia, 61
blood pressure, 10, 11, 14, 35, 45, 51-56, 63, 72, 86; diastolic, 49, 52; high, 3, 4, 6, 23, 28, 35, 40, 54-56, 71, 72, 80, 91, 93; low, 56, 105; systolic, 49, 52, 92
blood sugar level, 50, 54, 72
blood urea, 54
blood viscosity, 61
Body Mass Index (BMI), 26
Bonstetten, Charles Victor de, 68
bradyarrhythmias, 78
brain, 51, 54, 60, 101, 102
breathlessness, 4, 6-7, 55, 61, 107
bronchi, 62
bronchitis, 43, 61, 103
bronchospasm, 72
Burger's disease, 61
Business Week, 95
bypass surgery, 4, 21, 25, 36, 47, 75, 80, 88, 105, 107

cadmium, 60, 62
calcium channel blocker, 4, 6, 78, 79, 80
calories, 24, 27, 30, 35
cancer, 14, 21, 23, 25, 28, 30, 102; cervix, 61; lung, 22, 43, 61; oral cavity, 44, 61; stomach, 61; urinary bladder, 44, 61; voice box, 44, 61
Capital, 96
carbohydrate, 30, 35
carbon dioxide (CO_2), 60

carbon monoxide (CO), 60, 64, 65, 66; and cardiovascular system, 60-61
carboxyhaemoglobin, 60
cardiac cramps, 85
cardiac death, 18, 46, 61, 89
cardiac failure, 89
cardiac surgery, 82
cardiomyopathy, 3, 6, 31, 41
cardiopulmonary diseases, 64
cardiovascular disease, 26, 27, 30, 31, 35, 36, 58, 62, 63; in the elderly, 102, 103; prevention of, in the elderly, 107-108
cataract, 101, 104
Cato, 108
central nervous system, 101
cerebrovascular disease, 30, 31, 35, 36, 104
cervical spondylosis, 4
Charaka Samhita, 17, 20, 21, 24, 25, 41, 42, 48, 84, 85, 87, 92
Charaka Sutra, 85, 87, 89
Charka, 8, 88
Chaucer, 108
chemotherapy, 25
chest pain, 4-5
cholera, 98
cholesterol, 4, 8, 9, 26, 28, 29, 33, 35, 37, 38, 39, 45, 48, 50, 54, 71, 72-73, 78, 92; serum, 32, 33, 34, 35, 36
Cicere, De Senectuta, 99
claudication pain, 43, 44, 55, 100
clot, 45
cognitive disorders, 41
Collins, Mortimer, 20, 84
Computerised Tomography (CT), 55, 98
congenital cardiac defect, 5
congestive heart failure, 60, 79, 102, 103
constipation, 105
contraceptive pills, 47
coronary arterial tone, 93

Index

Coronary Artery Bypass Graft (CABG), 25
coronary artery disease, 4, 21, 22, 30, 31, 33, 34, 36, 42, 47, 58, 60, 61, 78, 80, 88, 89, 102, 105
corpulmonale, 46, 60, 103
cough, 56, 72, 79
cyanosis, 103

De Motus Cordis, 18
death, 15, 21, 36, 42, 43, 45, 74, 88, 101
dehydration, 51
dental caries, 31
dental problems, 101, 104
depression, 15, 105
diabetes, 3, 21, 22, 23, 31, 71, 78, 79
diarrhoea, 51
diet, 24, 27, 29, 30-40, 47, 54, 89, 94, 95; and longevity, 23, 26; balanced, 23, 27, 28; control, 33, 73; overeating, 23; related problems, 22, 31
dietary fibre, 30, 35
digestion, 87
digitalis, 6, 79
Diogenes, 90
Diogenes, Laertius, 90
diuretics, 6, 56, 79, 80, 105
dizziness, 61
drugs, 8, 21, 25, 34, 35, 42, 55, 56, 72, 76-83, 98, 104, 105, 107, 108
dust-storms, 65

Ebner, Maria Von, 10
Edwards, G., 99
Electrocardiogram (ECG), 54, 78, 93
electrolytes, 7, 56, 64, 80
Electron Microscopy, 98
emotions, 10, 14-15
endophrine, 49
environment: and heart diseases, 58-59; noise pollution, 63-66; pollution, 57-67

Epistular and Lucilium, 1
Eschenbach, 10
exhaustion, heat, 51
eyes, 54, 59

fatigue, 3, 4, 7, 55, 79
fats, 30, 31, 95; saturated, 33
Faust, 109
fevers, high, 51
foetal defects, 41
foetus, 44
folic acid, 9
formaldehyde, 61
Fortune, 96, 97
fungi, 60

Galen, 85
gall bladder disease, 4, 104; gastroenteritis, 56
gallstones, 23, 31
gangrene, 61
Gemfibrozil, 72
giddiness, 7, 105
Goethe, 109

haemoglobin, 60
Hales, Reverend Stephan, 86
Harvey, William, 18, 85
headache, 55, 61, 79
heart rate, 11, 14, 35, 45, 92
Heart to Heart-A Holistic Approach to Heart Care, 13
heart, 51, 60, 95, 100; and mind, 10-18; alarm signals of trouble, 3-7; attacks, 3, 8, 14, 17, 19, 26, 28, 29, 30-37, 41, 44, 45, 50, 51, 56, 63, 71-74, 75, 76, 78, 89, 92, 93, 101, 102, 103, 107; defects, 3-7; management, 1-9; muscle disease, 41, 51; problems, 1-9, 101-102; transplant, 25, 36, 99
heartbeat, 5, 11, 52, 73, 78, 85
Heberden, William, 86
hepatic lipase, 48

Hergeshemer, Joseph, 76
herpes, 4
High Density Lipoprotein (HDP), 26, 31, 46, 48, 50, 71, 73
Hippocrates, 22, 58
hoarseness of voice, 43
Holmer, Justice Oliver Wendell, 51, 108
Holter study, 78
homeostasis, 57
homoeopathy, 84
hormones, 10, 38
Horowitz, Dr. Steven, 95
How Old Are You?, 20
hydrocarbons, 60, 61, 66
hydrogencyamide, 61
hyperinsulnemia, 48
hypertension, 3, 19, 21, 22, 23, 29, 30, 31, 33, 35, 41, 45, 47, 48, 49, 51, 54, 55, 56, 58, 60, 62, 78, 79, 86, 92, 94, 102, 105, 107, 108; malignant, 46, 47; secondary, 55
hyperthyroidism, 3
hypokalemia, 105
hyponatremia, 105
hypotension, 8
hypothyroidism, 3, 7

impaired vision, 55
increased overall mortality, 41
industrial waste, 60
infections, 23
insulin, 48
Intensive Cardiac Care Unit (ICCU), 36, 104
intestinal disorders, 31
Intracardiac Cardioverter Defribrillators (ICD), 5, 106
irritability, 55
ischaemic heart disease, 62, 78

Journal (The), 100

Kamasutra, 106

kidneys, 51, 54, 59, 102, 104; failure, 51; disease, 55; transplant, 99
Kirpal, Prem, 13

Lancet (The), 94
laser, 21, 36, 99
lead, 60, 62, 64, 65
lethargy, lassitude, 7, 61, 78
lifestyle, 29, 32, 33, 36, 89; and longevity, 20-29; problems related to, 21-23; sedantary, 35, 48, 58, 87, 93
limbs, 80, 102
lipoprotein, 31
liver, 104; cirrhosis of, 41; transplant, 99
longevity, 18-19, 26-29, 42, 48, 49, 57-67, 68, 69, 84, 98-109; and diet, 23-26; lifestyle and, 20-29
Longfellow, 109
Low Density Lipoprotein (LDL), 31, 48, 50
Lucretius, 23
lungs, 59, 77, 80, 104; cancer of, 22, 43, 61; disease, 23, 60, 62, 103; transplant, 99

Magnetic CT scan, 98
Magnetic Resonance Imaging (MRI), 55, 98
meditation, 2, 27, 56, 72, 92, 93, 94, 95, 107
menopause, 53
mental relaxation, 2, 8, 11, 15-18, 24, 27, 49, 50, 56, 72, 74, 82, 89, 107; management, 73-74
mercury (Hg), 60
metabolism, 87; abnormalities, 45; process, 51
methane, 61
mind, and heart, 10-18
mitrichondrial level, 57
mitral valve, 6, 80
modern medicine, 98-109

Morituri Salutamus, 109
myocardial infarction, 4, 35, 45, 60, 61, 78, 86, 93, 104, 105
myocardial ischaemia, 93
myocardial revascularisation, 105
myocardium, 59, 62

Nanak, Guru, 22, 58
nausea, 79
neo-natology, 98
neoplasms, 62
nervous system, 37
neurohumoral activity, 19
neurological disorder, 41
New England Journal of Medicine, 48
nicotine, 60
nightmares, 72
Niranjananandji, Paramahansa, 91
nitrates, 4, 6, 47, 78, 79
nitric dioxide, 60
nitrogen dioxide (NO_2), 62, 64, 65, 66
non-cardiac surgery, 104-105
nutrition, 10, 24, 26-29, 101; over, 30, 58; under, 30

obesity, 21, 22, 23, 26-29, 31, 49, 71, 78, 92
oedema, 103
open heart surgery, 80
Ornish, Dean, 27, 89, 94, 95
osteoarthritis, 21, 23, 31, 101
ovaries, 101
Ozone (O_3), 60, 62, 64, 66

pacemakers, 5, 7, 78, 99, 102, 105-106
palpitation, 4, 5-6, 55
Patanjali, 90
Patent Ductus Arterious, 81
penicillin, 8
peptic ulcer, 4
pericarditis, 3

pericardium, 3
peripartum, 98
peripheral arterial diseases, 31, 46, 61
peripheral vasodilatory, 79
physical exercise, 1, 8, 24, 27, 28, 29, 38, 47-50, 52, 56, 71, 72, 73, 82, 87, 89, 95, 106, 107; aerobic, 89; isometric, 50; isotonic, 49, 50
polio, 98
pollution: air, 59-63; domestic, 67; environmental, 57-67; industrial, 66; noise, 63-67; vehicular, 66-67
Positron Emission Tomography (PET), 98
potassium, 7, 28, 30, 35, 40, 79
pregnancy, 43, 98
proarrhythmia, 78
prostrate, 101, 104
proteins, 27, 48, 59
pulmonary oedema, 62
pulmonary valve, 80
pulse rate, 10, 79

R-R interval, 93
R-R variability, 93
radiotherapy, 25
rate pressure product, 14, 49
rehabilitation, 71, 74-75, 106
renal splanchnic disease, 31
retirement, 100; and health, 100-101
rheumatic fever, 3, 8, 58
rheumatic heart disease, 3, 5, 8, 58
rheumatic valvular lesions, 102
Ribose Nucleic Acid (RNA), 59
Richter, Jean Paul, 57

salt, excess, 8, 23, 31, 35
secondary prophylaxis, 8
sedatives, 8, 49, 104
Seneca, 1

unsafe, 42; in elderly 106-107
Simonides, 108
skin, 14, 59
sleeplessness, 55
smallpox, 98, 101
Smith, Logan, 100
smog, 60
smoking, 1, 4, 8, 11, 21, 22, 23, 24, 29, 33, 40, 42-45, 58, 60, 61, 71-72, 78, 92, 93, 103, 107; anti campaigns, 62; passive, 43, 60, 61
sodium, 7, 28, 30
Sophocles, 108
starvation, 23
Statins, 72
stent, 4, 20, 36, 80, 81, 88, 89, 99, 105
stimulants, 8
stress, 10, 15, 18
stroke, 23, 28, 29, 31, 35, 41, 45, 47, 51, 101, 102, 103
sugar, excess, 23
sulphur dioxide (SO_2), 60, 62, 64, 65
Sushruta, 86
Sushruta-Nidan, 86
Suspended Particulate Matter (SPM), 60, 62, 64, 65
sweating, 55, 56, 103
syncope, 7, 86

tachyarrhythmias, 78, 103
thiazides, 35
thrombolytic therapy, 76
Thurlow, Edward Hovell, 98
thyrotoxicosis, 5
Time magazine, 94
toxins, 59
Traditional Wisdom and Heart Care, 27
tranquillisers, 49
Transmyocardial Laser Revascularisation (TMR), 5

tremors, 85
tricuspid valve, 80
triglycerides, 31, 46, 48, 50, 54, 73
trimetazidine, 79
tuberculosis, 3, 98
typhoid, 98

ulcers, 22
Ultrasonography, 55
unconsciousness, 7, 103
uric acid, 28, 54
uterus, 101, 105

valve replacements, 36
valvoplasty, balloon, 7
valvotomies, balloon, 80
varicose veins, 102
vasospasm, 60
vehicular emissions, 60, 62
ventricle, left, 6
ventricular septal defect, 81
venules, 86
Very Low Density Lipoprotein (VLDL), 31, 48
Victor, Charles, 107
virus, 60, 79
viscera, 102
vitamins, 8, 27, 28, 79
Vivekananda, 69
vomitting, 51

weakness, 3, 55, 56, 79
weight, 49; control, 8, 27, 56; over, 27, 73
White, Paul Dudly, 29
World Health Organisation (WHO), 24, 26, 41, 43, 57, 101; Day, 43; No Tobacco Day, 43, 63

Yoga Shastra, 90
Yoga, 27, 107; and the heart, 90-97; *Hatha Yoga*, 90; *Rajayoga*, 90